Disorders of Human Learning, Behavior, and Communication

Ronald L. Taylor and Les Sternberg
Series Editors

Miriam Cherkes-Julkowski   Nancy Gertner

Spontaneous Cognitive Processes in Handicapped Children

Springer-Verlag
New York Berlin Heidelberg
London Paris Tokyo

Miriam Cherkes-Julkowski, School of Education, Department of Educational Psychology, The University of Connecticut, Storrs, CT 06268, USA

Nancy Gertner, Gesell Institute, New Haven, CT 06511; Guilford Public Schools, Guilford, CT 06437, USA

Series Editors: Ronald L. Taylor and Les Sternberg, Exceptional Student Education, Florida Atlantic University, Boca Raton, Florida 33431-0991, USA

Library of Congress Cataloging-in-Publication Data
Cherkes-Julkowski, Miriam.
    Spontaneous cognitive processes in handicapped children / Miriam
Cherkes-Julkowski, Nancy Gertner.
        p.   cm. — (Disorders of human learning, behavior, and
communication)
    Bibliography: p.
    Includes index.
    1. Handicapped children—Education.   2. Learning.   3. Cognition in
children.   I. Gertner, Nancy.   II. Title.   III. Series.
LC4019.C47 1988
371.9—dc19   88-19062

Printed on acid-free paper.

Typeset by Publishers Service, Bozeman, Montana.
Printed and bound by R.R. Donnelley & Sons, Harrisonburg, Virginia.
Printed in the United States of America.

9 8 7 6 5 4 3 2 1

ISBN 0-387-96801-6 Springer-Verlag New York Berlin Heidelberg
ISBN 3-540-96801-6 Springer-Verlag Berlin Heidelberg New York

This book is dedicated to those who have tolerated our errors. Outstanding among them, not in order of the magnitude of their patience, are:

Liat, Rachel, and Klaus
Abigail, Matthew, Ben, and Joseph
Arthur and Fay Goldberg
Harry and Millie Levy
J.F. Cawley
Harris Kahn
A.J. Pappanikou
Adeline Theis
The children

Preface

The thinking that began this book arose out of some dissatisfaction with the relatively simplified, unidimensional model of development, which seems to have come to dominate the fields that address the needs of atypically developing children. It seemed impossible to us that developmental differences could explain the range of learning and coping styles we have seen and read about in children identified as mentally retarded, slow learning, learning disabled, nonhandicapped, and gifted. If a typical model of development did not account for what children with handicaps to learning could do, when they would do it, and how they would accomplish it, such a model was not likely to imply anything important about how to intervene with and help them. Unfortunately, when we first began to examine this problem, turning away from a developmental model for interpreting atypical behavior meant turning toward a behaviorist one. This was not very satisfying either. Again the assumptions were bothersome. We were expected to accept that all children, this time at all ages as well as with all kinds of diagnoses, learned in essentially the same way with perhaps some variation in rate, reactivity, reinforcement preferences, and, according to more liberal applications, expectancy. In our search for a more satisfying view of the atypical learner, we were lucky to be lost at the moment when cognitive psychology and systems theory were being found.

We have started from the assumption that a child who is atypical by virtue of a disorder in learning has his or her own idiosyncratic nature, which is not irrelevant as we consider the child's present status and how we should provide instruction. There must have been some initial reason for the atypicality. Whether that initial difference persists or not, it must certainly have influenced each successive acquisition and reorganization. Perhaps the child has gone down "the road less traveled" and has had different options for subsequent paths because of it. It did not seem to make sense to adhere to an instructional style that assumed the road to be the same, only the mileage different. Instead we tried to uncover what qualitative differences among groups of differently labeled children, or simply different children, might be. This meant abandoning the frames for deciding what was good thinking, what were effective strategies, and how one could get more of them. What is presented in some of our earlier publications and in this book is an effort to understand how atypical learners might have organized themselves for the effort of learning and how we might, as instructors, adapt to that organization rather than insist that they adapt to ours.

The first three chapters in this book elaborate on the basis for our belief that it is important to go beyond a linear, universal model of development into the idiosyncratic organization and reorganizations of the learner who is not able to shift his or her course of development to meet the one that we have come to expect. In Chapter 4, we found it necessary to explain why it was so important to delve into the world of social cognition to find a procedure for understanding how children think and learn. The remainder of the book is devoted to the research we have done in the effort to understand what atypical children do spontaneously and effectively in their efforts to learn. Finally, we have presented our findings and some suggestions for using them in schools to the advantage of the atypical child.

We have attempted to raise some questions about the utility of assuming that there are universally "good" strategies for learning and therefore teaching. We have not yet gathered together the hubris (or chutzpah, if you prefer) to suggest firm solutions.

Miriam Cherkes-Julkowski
Nancy Gertner

Contents

1
Cogito Ergo Sum

A round man cannot be expected to fit into a square hole right away. He must have time to modify his shape.

Montramps abroad, 1897

Stereotypes about "good learning" and "effective instruction" have begun to give way to a regard for the idiosyncrasies that each learner brings to each situation. This change has taken place in the context of an increasing interest in cognitive psychology. The effect on special education is only now beginning to be felt (Cawley, 1985; Reid & Hresko, 1981). Until now the understanding of handicaps to learning has been rooted in developmental and behavioral psychology. The developmental view has provided a standard according to which growth could be measured. Once a child's accomplishments along developmental continua had been identified, his or her disorder could be defined in terms of relative delays in one or more areas (e.g., in reading, language, or both). Behavioral psychology provided the solution by establishing procedures to evoke performance at those levels not yet attained.

The cognitive view has added a new emphasis: the role of processes or strategies in thinking and learning. Disorders might be found in any of those functions associated with effective learning. There has been a rich literature attempting to identify those processes that facilitate learning in various areas. For example, efficient auditory memory has been valued as an effective strategy for decoding in reading (Vellutino & Steger, 1975). Elaborative strategies have been valued as a means for comprehending and remembering new information. There has been some discussion of particular strategies best suited to particular tasks (Brown, 1982; Jenkins, 1979). Most recently there has been an effort to understand the role of metacognitive strategies in thinking and learning.

What typifies all of this literature has been the attempt to identify how competent learners function and to simulate this experience for handicapped children. Such a model poses at least two problems. The first is that even competent learners are not free from errors. Their successful strategies do not exist in isolation. Their successes are embedded in a pattern and history of unsuccessful or partially successful attempts. To isolate only those strategies associated most closely with success is to devise a very superficial if not artificial view of competent cognition. The second problem is that children whose cognitive processes are impaired may manifest a set of strategies associated with success quite different from that of unimpaired, intact children (Cherkes-Julkowski, Gertner, & Norlander, 1986).

A simple technique of judging impaired learning against a template of effective processes may be insufficient. The pattern of strategies used by subgroups of handicapped learners must be assessed in its own light. Even a slight impairment in a single area can cause otherwise typically functioning areas to readjust. Just as a weak left leg might require an abnormal posture for successful ambulation, "correct" processing can assume a different posture in disordered learners.

Developmental Equivalence

Special education has tended to uphold the traditional view of development (Gesell & Amatruda, 1947; Piaget & Inhelder, 1969), which maintains that all children, regardless of culture or competence, progress through the same milestones. As a result, it is common to see developmental scales (*Battelle Developmental Inventory*, 1986; Gesell & Amatruda, 1947; Frankenburg, Dodds, & Fandal, 1975) used first to identify delayed rates of growth and then to provide the objectives for intervention (Furuno et al., 1979; Lillie, 1975). The assumption is that individual differences lie in the rate of progress through these steps and in the highest level ultimately achieved (Wishart, 1987). The concept of mental or developmental age is based in this kind of thinking. The suggestion is that a child who has achieved, for example, the final stages of object permanence (Uzgiris & Hunt, 1975) is equivalent to any other child 24 months of age. Whether that child is in reality 18 or 36 months old is, according to this view, relatively unimportant. The effects of more or less actual experience, as reflected by chronological age and the equality of experience as measured by ability or rate of development, is considered insignificant.

At later ages the developmental equivalence view takes two primary forms. At a very basic level, curricula for children with handicaps are designed to be compatible with curricula in the mainstream. Curriculum guidelines and objectives assume the position of developmental milestones during the period in which the child is in school. The procedure is essentially the same: expect the same pattern of growth at a slower rate and expect a lower endpoint. In a more literal application of the developmental model, objectives for children with learning disorders are typically task-analyzed. The task analysis takes on the stature of a developmental continuum and, again, children of a wide range of backgrounds and abilities are assumed to progress in similar fashions, albeit at different rates, through the continuum. In the same way that developmental continua are used as both assessment and curriculum devices, the steps in task analysis dictate curriculum objectives as well as items for assessing the progress of the child. The latter form a criterion-referenced test (CRT).

To use a criterion-referenced instrument, the examiner or teacher takes the child through the steps leading toward a given final objective. Each step at which the child is able to perform adequately, or pass, represents a skill that has been acquired. The purpose of criterion-referenced testing is to take the child through the gradations of the task to identify exactly what he or she can or cannot do. When the level is reached at which the child can no longer perform, the typical interpretation is that this is the exact level at which to begin instruction. One of the other supposed virtues of the CRT, then, is that it contains an approach to assessment as well as an entire set of objectives for instruction (Gronlund, 1976).

What Develops?

The question concerning CRTs is the same as in the case of developmental scales: Namely, does either describe growth in both handicapped and nonhandicapped populations? Since the CRT aims at identifying the exact level and content of a child's growth up to this point, an effective, valid CRT would have to reflect an empirically supported developmental, hierarchical sequence of steps. This goal is almost unattainable given the state of our understanding of developmental processes. Even the most widely substantiated hierarchies of development, upon which CRTs such as Uzgiris and Hunt's Ordinal Scales of Psychological Development (1975) (an adaptation of Piaget's theory) have been based, have not been made to withstand the more critical tests of developmental validity such as a Guttman analysis (Uzgiris & Hunt, 1987).

Despite the strong investment in developmental theory as a basis for special education, in the past decade the very concept of qualitative, hierarchically organized changes over time have met with considerable challenge (Chi, 1978; Fagan, 1982; Fodor, 1975). Traditional views of development (Gesell & Amatruda, 1947; Piaget & Inhelder, 1969) emphasize the epigenetic nature of maturation and the role of experience in triggering the evolution of increasingly higher-level cognitive structures with which a learner can view and operate on experiences. What develops, in theory, is the quality of the structures available for processing information. Once a higher-level structure has evolved, the learner is capable of learning and thinking about higher-level, more complex, more abstract ideas. Accordingly, infants and young children are capable only of concrete knowledge, no abstractions. As they mature and have challenging (disequilibrating) experiences, higher-level programs for processing information become available. In the Piagetian view, this evolves as a result of the assimilation/accommodation process.

As procedures for studying thinking become more sophisticated (Fagan, 1982; Zelazo, 1982), evidence for higher and higher levels of cognitive functioning are being uncovered at earlier and earlier ages. It is not uncommon to talk about the competent infant. Evidence of analogical reasoning (Caron & Caron, 1981), abstract thinking (Baillergon & Graber, 1987), and number concept (Strauss & Curtis, 1981), as well as the structures that enable these kinds of thinking, have been found within the first year of life. Fodor (1975) is of a similar opinion, that structures for higher-level thinking are present from the beginning. He derives his conclusion based on logical contradiction within developmental theory rather than on empirical evidence as do those previously cited:

What *couldn't* happen . . . is that the device (cognitive/language system) uses the available conceptual system to *learn* the more powerful (developmentally advanced) one. That is, what couldn't happen is that it gets from stage one to stage two by anything that we would recognize as a computational procedure (in the Gagne sense of concept learning or any other information processing model). In short, trauma might do it; so might maturation. Learning won't . . . . What has been argued is, in effect, this: If the mechanism of concept learning is the projection and confirmation of hypotheses (and what else *could* it be), then there is a sense in which there can be no such thing as learning a new concept (Fodor, 1975, p. 93, 95).

Neo-Piagetian or post-Piagetian thinking offers some alternative explanations for what develops. Although there are several different neo-Piagetian positions about development, all agree that the structures for abstract, higher-level thinking are present from birth. If this is true, the question remains, what changes with growth from infancy to adulthood? Neo-Piagetian explanations to this question might be classified broadly into three different frameworks: capacity theory (Case, 1985); knowledge-based/constraint theories (Chi, 1985; Nelson, 1987); and neofunctionalism (Fodor, 1981; Rosch, 1983).

Capacity Theory

Capacity Theory (Case, 1978, 1985; Pascual-Leone, 1976) modifies the traditional Piagetian view of development by suggesting that ways of thinking do not change over time, but one's capacity for dealing with information does. Younger children and, by implication. those with impairments to learning have reduced M power (Pascual-Leone, 1976). The term *M power* refers to the number of mental schemes for processing information that can be activated simultaneously. It is similar to notions of short-term memory or digit span as measured on the Wechsler Intelligence Scale for Children—Revised (WISC-R) (Wechsler, 1974). In all persons, capacity for attending to and maintaining information in working memory is limited. Space has been reported to allow initially for two or three bits of information to be processed at a time (Case, 1978; Chi, 1978; Pascual-Leone, 1976). Children through the ages of 3 and 4 years are characterized by this kind of capacity. Span increases with age, presumably as a result of maturation or general experience (Pascual-Leone, 1976), until Miller's (1956) "magic number 7 plus or minus 2" is reached during adulthood. Increased space or capacity allows for a greater amount of information to be processed simultaneously. Since complex ideas require the manipulation of a number of bits of information, the recognition of patterns, themes, and variations, as well as complexity, depends on adequate capacity. Adults, therefore, are capable of appreciating a greater degree of complexity not because they have more advanced, qualitatively different operational structures, but because they can consider greater amounts of information in a greater number of interrelationships at a given time than can children.

Case (1978) has described the evolution of number conservation in terms of capacity and M power rather than in the traditional Piagetian way of changes in underlying cognitive structures. The capacity view argues that until a child can process information from the perceptual field ("This string of M&M's looks longer") simultaneously with information about number ("There are 5 in the shorter string and only 4 in the longer one") as well as recognize and cope with the conflict, he or she will not be able to cope with conservation problems. The assumption remains, however, that the same child is cognitively capable of formulating concepts about number and about the perceptual field, and can recognize conflict as long as each is dealt with independently and within capacity limitations. The implication is that number concept per se is not dependent on cognitive structures, which evolve at the time at which conservation is mastered. Instead, the cognitive structures are already present and are awaiting great enough M power to be used in achieving thorough number concept.

Strauss and Curtis (1981) have studied number concept in infancy. They have established that infants can recognize number concept in a conservation-like task as early as the 10th month. Infants, however, can only make equivalence judgments about the quantities of 2 and 3 and sometimes 4, never beyond this amount. The match between early numerosity and basic capacity is quite convincing. Interestingly, Spitz (1966) reports that children and adults with mental retardation are limited to a span of three bits of information. Capacity does not seem to grow with age or experience. More will be said about the nature of capacity increase and whether it is real (structural) or metaphorical (an apparent outgrowth of improved ability to maximize a finite amount of capacity).

Capacity is consumed not only by the amount of information being processed but also by higher-level metacognitive functions concerned with processing that information (Case, 1985; Schiffrin & Dumais, 1981). It is a continual trade-off, then, between the allotment of capacity to either of these two functions: information processing and the decision of when and how to perform which processes. Higher-level functions include strategies for attending to and imposing meaning on information such as clustering, elaboration, or other mnemonic devices as well as executive control functions that examine task demands, select, plan, and monitor appropriate strategies, or information processing devices. Development or enhancement of the system is seen as growth in the ability to maximize the use of limited capacity.

Since capacity at any given point in development is a finite system, the challenge is to move information in and out of working memory as quickly as possible. The process calls up the image of juggling or of attempting to ward off a rush of overflowing water by capturing it in an 8 oz container, emptying, refilling, and the like. The goal is rapid access to information strategies and to previously learned relevant contexts, efficient execution of these, and ultimately reduced residence time in the working memory store. Functional increases in capacity, then, can be achieved from several different sources. One that has received some attention from Case as well as other researchers in the field of learning disabilities is automaticity (Samuels, 1987; Schiffrin & Dumais, 1981; Swanson, 1987). Automatic processing is compared to controlled processing:

Controlled processing requires attention and decreases the system capacity that is available for other processing. Automatic processing does not necessarily demand processing resources, freeing the system for higher-level processing and alternative control processing (Schiffrin & Dumais, 1981, p. 111).

For a skill or process to function at an automatic level, then, it must be triggered at an implicit level and with little or no need for mediation. A major goal of schooling in the early years is to bring computational skills in math and decoding skills in reading to an automatic level. Once this is accomplished the higher-level functions of mathematical problem solving and advanced operations, as well as higher-level reading comprehension processes, can recruit the attention they need. In the absence of automaticity with lower-level functions, attention is diluted across too many dimensions and capacity does not allow for consideration of higher-level issues. Lack of automaticity in lower-level functions is an attribute typically associated with children and adults with learning disorders (Perfetti & Hogaboam, 1975). Learning-disabled and -delayed children are frequently described as having slow reaction time and as being neurologically disorganized. In some children, disintegrated, nonautomatic responding is possibly based in a central nervous system dysfunction. In addition, initial lack of automaticity with very basic skills becomes a block to the development of automatic functions at higher levels.

A further risk to effective automaticity in learning-disabled students is their tendency to develop faulty or cumbersome algorithms or procedures for operating on information. Consider the case of a child referred for math problems in the beginning of the third grade. She has assumed that adding from left to right is a valid procedure. As soon as two-digit numbers are introduced, perhaps at the end of the first or beginning of the second grade, she applies her left-to-right procedure. Since renaming is not required at the initial stages, she receives positive feedback 100% of the time for her approach. Eventually, renaming will be introduced, but probably along with some of the easier examples where no renaming is required. At this point the student is intermittently reinforced for her procedure, probably more often than not. After more than two school years of extensive drilling with this procedure, the purpose of which is to develop automaticity, a strong, automatic or nearly automatic counterproductive strategy has been inadvertently trained. The existence of counterproductive strategies, be they procedural (such as left-to-right addition), affective (such as learned helplessness), or behavioral (such as acting out or cheating), becomes a further obstacle to learning. What is more, such strategies create a dynamic that is qualitatively different from the one originally intended by the instructional design.

Efficient processing in the form of increased capacity can be further facilitated by the automatic use of information-reducing strategies. Children with handicaps to learning are notorious for their deficiencies in the use of strategies for managing and remembering information. They seem unable to evoke appropriate strategies or any strategies at all in the face of task demands (Cherkes-

Julkowski et al., 1986). Competent learners use a range of strategies to give greater meaning to new information such as elaboration, visual imagery, or key-word or peg-word procedures. They tend to use mnemonic devices to group or condense information, such as developing acronyms to represent strings of infor-mation (FOIL—first, outer, inner, last—to represent an abbreviated approach to solving quadratic equations) or using rhymes to remember strings of words or numbers. They might cluster information based on some common physical or categorical attribute, they might simply rehearse new information repeatedly until it is automatic. All of these procedures seem to reduce stress on working memory capacity by chunking information into smaller units (Miller, 1956), by associating it with previously learned information and thereby coming to terms with meaning and releasing the demand for continued attention, or by making responses automatic. There is extensive literature confirming that learning-disabled and -delayed children or adults are less likely to use any of these stra-tegies; however, they can be trained to do so (Brown, Bransford, Ferrara, & Campione, 1983). As a result, they remember as well as their mental-age peers. Nevertheless, no training has been completely successful in assisting handi-capped learners in invoking these strategies spontaneously (Cherkes-Julkowski et al., 1986). The result is the repeated finding that learning-disabled and men-tally retarded students do not achieve an attention span of greater than 3 units. They fail to achieve automaticity and are frequently overwhelmed by the demands of the situation.

Knowledge Base

Traditional developmental theory depends largely on the assumption that older persons are capable of more complex thinking than younger ones. Although this is a generally valid proposition, the question remains, what, if anything, develops to make higher-level thinking available to older learners/thinkers. Capacity theories argue that space and M power increase. It is then possible to deal with greater amounts of information at a time. Since complexity is defined by amount of information and intricacies of relationships, sufficient span would be necessary for its appreciation. Knowledge-base theories suggest that space might be an indirect explanation for the growth of complexity. What truly develops over time is neither structures for operating on the world nor the architecture of span (Pascual-Leone, 1976), but the size and interconnectedness of the knowledge store (Chi, 1985). Young children are "universal novices" (Chi, 1978). Their sparse knowledge is stored as a limited number of nodes or data points. Their limited experience has created fewer links between nodes. With repeated and varied exposure to situations, more nodes are created as well as more connections between them.

Chi has compared child experts in chess to adult novices (1978) as well as child dinosaur experts to child novices (1985). In both comparisons, experts were able to remember more about the subject area and remembered in larger as well as more integrated chunks. The more expert the chess player or dinosaur maven, the more connections there were among nodes in the area. In comparison with adult novices, children were capable of a greater memory span as well as more efficient recall and greater complexity. The cognitive abilities for appreciating complexity, then, are clearly not dependent on chronological age, but rather on experience and previous learning.

As Chi (1985) develops the idea of the relationship between number of nodes stored and multiplicity of connections among them, she describes what she identifies as *knowledge networks*. Another metaphor for the integration of knowledge sites might be that of a road map. The greater number of interconnections or throughways on a road map, the greater the efficiency of access. Speed of access is of very real importance in the light of limited capacity and the need to reduce allocation of attention to retrieval processes. If a novel event occurs, an object needs to be identified or a problem solved, the likelihood of recognizing some aspect of the novel situation is increased less by the number of bits of information stored than by the possibility of moving between those bits in a search for some relevant frame or frames.

Well-integrated road systems are effective in increasing efficiency in the form of leading to frames that can elaborate on or impose meaning on novel stimuli. The benefits of such a system are twofold. Rapid access to meaning reduces the need to allocate limited resources to maintaining information in working memory and, thus, in effect, allows for greater capacity. Access to relevant frames also facilitates integration of this new information bit into the existing long-term store, thereby increasing the potential of the entire system. Well-integrated knowledge networks or systems are more likely to allow for flexibility in thinking. The road map metaphor works here as well. If one knows how to get to Denver only by way of Boston, a trip from Tallahassee is likely to be too burdensome to undertake. If the trip is taken repeatedly over time, the opportunity to learn further subconnections is diminished due, at least in part, to lack of alternative routes. The taken path becomes increasingly dominant as a response mode until it is automatized and perhaps rigidly evoked as the "solution" to getting to Denver, perhaps from San Francisco as well.

What develops according to this view is the richness and complexity of the knowledge structure. With increased linkages, the likelihood for adapting previous learning to novel situations is greater. The sheer probability of finding some association between the to-be-learned event and existing information within the network is greater. The association ultimately made is more meaningful because it is better connected. Chi (1985) has demonstrated that larger and better-integrated knowledge networks functionally increase capacity through rapid access to meaning and, therefore, reduced need to exhaust limited attentional and working memory resources. At this point the learner can experience the benefits of increased capacity as described by capacity theory: increased complexity of thinking. Since young children are usually less informed than older children or adults, the progression of increased competence appears to be developmental. But, as Chi (1978) has demonstrated in her chess studies, young child experts have the cognitive capability of thinking in a more advanced form than adult novices.

The quality of the knowledge network influences generalization, transfer of learning, or more broadly, problem solving. Persons with retardation are described as having few fall-back strategies and failing to recognize the need for subtle shifts in strategy application (Cherkes-Julkowski et al., 1986). This is perhaps most vivid in the area of social competence. Although it is possible to train moderately and severely retarded adults to greet others in a socially desirable way (e.g., "Good morning, how are you?"), the behavior becomes maladaptive if the other person is a stranger and prefers not to communicate. No response is acceptable repeatedly across all situations. Training that suggests that a single response might suffice contributes to rigidity by failing to create several scenarios that call up different subsystems within the "greet others" knowledge subroutine.

Learning-disabled youngsters and adults also have difficulty in the face of a need for flexibility. They are likely to remain passive (Wong, 1980), to say they do not know how to do that one and wait for someone to show them how, or to assume that a single procedure can be used to solve all, even vaguely similar, problems. So, in a three-digit plus three-digit addition problem,

$$452$$
$$+\ 321$$

the answer is figured as "2 + 1 is 3 and 5 is 8, and 2 is 10 . . ." until the answer 17 is achieved. To extend the road map metaphor, when asked to go to San Francisco, the solver can only set out on the path from Tallahassee, through Boston, and end in Denver. Ironically, many children with learning disorders do the cognitive equivalent of this and do not realize where they are going until they are stuck in Denver.

The problem is not limited to handicapped or young persons. Doctoral students just prior to their defense inevitably ask what will happen if they are asked a question for which they do not have an answer. They seem surprised, and relieved, to be told that they would be certain to know something that would bear on the question and produce some interpretation or analysis. It seems to be a new notion that there is not one pathway from problem to solution, but many.

Whatever rigidity exists in handicapped children manifests itself almost from birth. Loveland (1987) describes the difference in the play of Down's syndrome and nonhandicapped infants. She, among others, has found that children with Down's syndrome engage in more stereotyped, repetitive, nonexploratory play than children without handicaps. In her study of children with mental ages from 16 to 32 months, Loveland investigated the abilities of the handicapped and the nonhandicapped to find things seen reflected in a mirror. She found that nonhandicapped children tended to use a greater variety of strategies to locate the reflected object: turning to look in the wrong direction, leaving the room, or looking behind the mirror. She describes these as "active but incorrect strategies" (p. 934). In contrast, the children with Down's syndrome displayed a fixed unelaborated search pattern. More will be said about the virtue of incorrect strategies in the following chapter.

Wishart (1987) finds similar differences in learning processes between preschoolers with Down's syndrome and those who are nonhandicapped. Wishart's nonhandicapped 3- to 4-year-olds were relatively quick to figure out where an object was hidden in one of the most advanced Piagetian object permanence tasks. All children were asked to do the task six times. By the third time, the nonhandicapped children had responded correctly and had begun to "tease" the examiner by smiling and making contrived incorrect responses. The children with Down's syndrome mastered the task as well. They, however, displayed little interest in the just-mastered task and instead preferred to operate at the next developmental level. The handicapped population, then, does not provide itself with a "playing around" period, which Wishart (1987) suggests is necessary to consolidate already mastered learning. Through consolidation the newly acquired skill or concept becomes integrated into the existing knowledge structure. Perhaps the initial and persistent difference between the nonhandicapped and the handicapped in how they learn lies in the ability to provide elaborations rich enough to sustain interest and, therefore, attention after habituation to an event.

Krakow and Kopp (1983) have also presented evidence for early differences between infants with Down's syndrome and nonhandicapped populations. Despite the fact that handicapped and nonhandicapped children sustain attention for a comparable amount of time during an independent play session, the quality of how attention is deployed is different in a nontrivial way. Handicapped children are inclined to attend to a given object or person and to focus on it to the exclusion of other events in the immediate environment. In contrast, nonhandicapped children would glance away from the target activity more frequently. The advantages to well-deployed attention are clear in terms of incidental learning, ability to maintain contact with caregivers for the sake of refueling, and, in general, access to enriched experiences. The implications for the amount and interconnectivity of information in the knowledge store are profound. Not only does each experience produce more information for the knowledge store, but each bit of information has multiplicative effects in the potential to learn about further events. The vastness of these differences cannot be equated through formulas that equate the mental ages of handicapped and nonhandicapped children.

Qualitative differences during the early stages of development, then, have direct implications for the evolution of the knowledge structure. At each experience it seems that nonhandicapped persons have had a wider exposure. Although not all forms of exploration lead directly to solution of the problem at hand, each attempt brings in some information that enriches the knowledge network. If each experience is more stripped down for the child with handicaps, there are multiplicative effects on the knowledge store. From the beginning, the handicapped child is set upon a trajectory that is qualitatively different from that of a typically developing child. Chapter 3 goes into some detail about the nature of qualitative differences and their effects on learning.

Neonativism / Neofunctionalism

A theory of development that adheres to qualitative, structural changes over time may not describe growth even for nonhandicapped populations. The contemporary, neonativist picture (Case, 1985; Fagan, 1982; Fodor, 1975) consists of an infant born with all of the abilities that he or she will ever acquire for processing information. This position differs from Piaget's notions in profound ways. Contrary to traditional developmental theory, it is argued that logical propositional forms of analysis (schemata) do not change over time and do not govern mental operations. Neofunctionalism (Rosch, 1983) argues that learning and concept formation is not characterized by explicit, logical analysis of the kind presumed to comprise Piaget's schemata. Instead, both children and adults represent events according to more holistic analogue models, initially unanalyzed, primarily as events exist in the external world. Prototypical events become organizers or referents for evolving categories and relationships (Rosch, 1983). The neofunctionalist view sees the learner as one who is impressed by the relationships and systematic covariance of real-world events. The learner appreciates, for example, that animals with wings are likely to have feathers (Rosch, 1983). Frames for understanding the world, then, are not determined primarily by internally evolving structures. Instead, they are imprinted by the structures that exist externally. A theory that does not acknowledge the primacy of internally derived structures certainly has no need for explaining their qualitative changes with age. Nelson (1987) takes a more moderate position. She argues that perhaps language introduces the single qualitative shift in development. Language introduces the means for cognitive control processes, thereby allowing for conscious analysis of information and the thinking process itself (metacognition).

In all of these views, the dominant theme is that the traditional model of development does not describe growth for either handicapped or nonhandicapped populations. Children seem to learn in the same way as adults from the infant period forward. What changes over time is the quantity and quality of stored experience. As more knowledge exists, as greater experience with each concept is accrued, events become increasingly differentiated at the same time that they become increasingly embedded into an integrated network. Ultimately, higher-level, metacognitive control can be realized, which allows for even greater efficiency. This process is not developmental but is the result of the specific effects of learning (Liben, 1987) within systems theory (see Chapter 2).

Implications for Atypical Populations

Special education, however, has relied heavily on the developmental metaphor. Children with mental retardation are described as having pervasive *delays*. In terms of treatment they are taken to be similar to nonhandicapped children with the same mental age. In order to be identified as learning disabled, a child or adult must demonstrate a *delay* in one or more of eight specified areas of achievement. The language of delay creates the expectation for educators as well as parents that these children are the same in one or more areas as nonhandicapped children. Once they achieve a "milestone," handicapped children have conquered the same things in the same ways as those without handicaps. There is even the implication that a delay allows for the possibility of catching up. Children who manifest language disorders during their first 3 years provide an interesting example. Although many ultimately manage to use rules of syntax and to develop vocabulary, word-finding problems, circumlocutions, and various forms of verbal apraxia are likely to persist through adolescence and adulthood. This is not to imply that such persons are forever dysfunctional. It is to state, however that initial differences provide the need for compensatory devices that are achieved through an atypical organization of processes governing language or the process in question. This initial structure, once established, is that which provides the context, the potential, for further growth.

From the perspective of systems theory, development is a result of the dynamic transaction among various subsystems or structures. To extend the example of the language-disordered child, the initial atypical adaptation is made at the expense of a "typical" one and at the expense of other potential adaptations. The paths not taken become abilities that are nor incorporated into this, or potentially other, reorganizations. Since each subsystem alters the character of the entire system, the initial adaptation to language problems alters the entire organization and developmental pathway of the individual. There are children, for example, whose receptive linguistic competence is appropriate for their age and ability. At the same time, despite good pragmatic communication through gesture and sign and adequate oral musculature, their expressive abilities are quite limited. The initial etiology might have included emotional disturbance, dyspraxia, or problems in organizing complex responses. In addition to the initial cause and its unique long-term effects, the atypical adaptation in the form of manual sign and gesture becomes a momentum for development in itself. A child who expresses herself in this way is likely to fail to use verbal labels for coding and storing semantic information. The direct outcome might include a more diffusely organized semantic store, less efficient word retrieval even at a recognition level, and ultimately impaired verbal mediation processes for the purpose of cognitive control. There may be indirect effects as well. It is likely that such a child will need to or will be naturally inclined to develop imagery as a primary form of representation. It has been recognized that imagery is primarily a right-brain function (Popper & Eccles, 1977), which requires the simultaneous (Kaufman & Kaufman, 1983) processing of information in an implicit, unanalyzed form. If this tendency becomes strong enough it has the potential for many positive outcomes, but also for overriding more explicit, sequential, analytical processes required for early reading and math skill acquisition.

Ironically, the more talented a child becomes in compensating for an initial disorder, the more ingrained might become the disorder, with its present as well as potential atypical adaptations. Problems in any domain (e.g., language), then, relate to, magnify, or modify functioning in others (e.g., mnemonic strategies, behavior control, reading, math, executive function, interpersonal relationships, and so on). It is possible, in fact probable, that some of the resulting compensatory behaviors resulting from initial delays or disorders appear maladaptive as well. A vivid example is the prolonged, perseveration-like play behavior of blind children, which has been described as an extended period of autism (Fraiberg, 1977). Another, and in our view more plausible, explanation is that extended and repetitive play is truly exploratory for the child with visual impairment. Visual perception allows for a rapid three-dimensional representation of an object in all of its transformation (Cooper & Shepard, 1973). To gain all of this information haptically takes considerable time and sampling of the object in order to reconstruct a comparable representation. All atypical behaviors, then, are not necessarily maladaptive. Likewise, individual problems or behaviors cannot be treated individually without disturbing the balance of the entire coping mechanism (Stolzenberg & Cherkes-Julkowski, 1987).

There are neurological correlates of atypical adaptations as well. These exist in addition to and to some degree biologically independent of any initial damage or dysfunction. Patterns of neural connectivity are sculpted through active involvement with the environment in the form of the elimination and simultaneous selective retention of synapses (Goldman-Rakic, 1987). In this way each brain derives its own organization. Studies of sensory deprivation in animals during early development indicate resulting impairment in the processing of information from the deprived channels, for example, visual information processing when animals are reared in darkness (Greenough, Black, & Wallace, 1987). Interestingly, prolonged visual deprivation seems to affect the perception of *relationships* among the elements of a visual display rather than the ability to cope with more or less discrete bits of information (Tees, 1979). Although some recovery of visual information processing in deprived kittens has been effected, approximately half of the neurons do not recover, and it remains impossible to orient to stimuli across the midline (Sherman, 1977).

Externally controlled experience per se does not explain differential brain organization. How experience is actively processed is far more relevant (Held & Hein, 1963). Despite similar exposure to auditory stimuli, the auditory cortex becomes larger in animals who have been visually deprived (Ryugo, Ryugo, Glubus, & Killackey, 1975). Experience and the way it is actively processed within the context of the existing organization is a critical component in the determination of the pattern of neural connections (Greenough et al., 1987). Children can have atypical experiences due either to deprivation or to internally driven strengths and weaknesses. Our child, who does not use spoken language for verbal expression and possibly for coding experience, is an example of the latter. Each of these experiences with neural organization and reorganization (Witelson, 1987) has its effects on the current and potential status of the system.

"Typical" Development

Given idiosyncratic reorganizations dependent upon individual experiences as well as potential, it is difficult to conceptualize what might be typical about development or growth. It is perhaps more productive to view typicality as a band of possibilities, which when exceeded raises concern about an individual's capacity to make further appropriate adaptations. It is interesting to note that the measurement of cognitive abilities has come to adopt the latter position. Although the original Stanford–Binet Intelligence Scale assumed a developmental model and produced a developmental score, the newly revised Stanford–Binet (Thorndike, Hagen, & Sattler, 1986), as well as other relatively recent measures (Kaufman & Kaufman, 1983) of cognitive abilities, uses a deviation formula for describing abilities.

Dunst (1980) has called for another approach to the measurement, identification, and understanding of atypical populations. It is not enough, he argues, to rely on scores that reflect deviations form a normative model of development. That a child's functioning is significantly discrepant from the norm says little about the nature of the atypicality or how it interacts with other relatively weak or strong domains. The quality of an atypical child's abilities would be better expressed as a profile of performance across relevant domains. The psychometric manifestation of this approach would be to produce norms for subgroups of disordered populations based on patterns of strengths and weaknesses across a series of abilities. Profile analysis of this sort would suggest something about the internal organization of types of disorders as well as about the individual and, thus, how instruction could be made to fit within this context. In this way it would be possible to begin a systematic approach to identifying subtypes of learning disabilities.

Instruction Based on a Developmental Versus Difference Model

Most of instruction for learning-disordered populations is based not only in the developmental model, but also in the assumption that disordered individuals are basically the same as nonhandicapped learners, only slower in a given area or in all areas and possibly reach a different endpoint. The assumption is that development is a hierarchy of steps. All children ascend the ladder in the same way. Such a position does not acknowledge the role of initially differential organization and later idiosyncratic reorganizations, nor does it recognize that children with initial differences will evolve alternative pathways for learning and living (J. B. Stolzenberg, personal communication). Initial qualitative differences, then, exist in the fabric of abilities and achievements. They provide a qualitatively different frame from which to develop further. In the developmental tradition, individualization takes the form of deciding where on a continuum one child might be and targeting instruction toward those objectives not yet achieved. Individualization of this kind typically attempts to design good criterion-referenced testing and good instruction at the appropriate level. Blankenship (1978) reports the outcome of her attempts to apply this approach to children with math disabilities. Eighty-eight percent of her population was "cured" in an extraordinary average rate of 38 seconds of instruction. Blankenship concludes that the remaining 12% who were not correctable using her model were truly disabled learners for whom qualitatively different forms of instruction would be necessary.

It would be unproductive to persist in "good instruction" with the population represented by Blankenship's 12%. Davis (personal communication) has described this colorfully as the Vietnam solution: If it doesn't work, do more of it. In our view, what is indicated is an attempt to discover what the nature of the learner's organization of previous, related experience seems to be, how this generates specific interpretations of events, and to tailor instruction to work from this perspective forward.

If development has been set off on an atypical path, it is possible that it will include a different progression of steps and atypical approaches to their attainment. Fraiburg (1977) makes this point about the development of blind children, whom she describes as having a prolonged period of autistic play. A strict developmental approach might proceed to supplant this level with the next level of appropriate (i.e., typical) behavior. A more forgiving but still developmental approach might tolerate it for some time, but ultimately attempt to herd the child's actions back on an upwardly moving "correct" developmental course. Intervention that follows from a different view would be likely to attempt to recognize in what appears to be perseverative behavior anything that might constitute meaningful interaction, albeit atypical. Visual perception allows for immediate knowledge of the three-dimensional properties of an object and all its rotations. Without it, the learner needs to explore each aspect of an object from all angles to achieve a similarly complete awareness. Clearly, knowing an object is going to be a lengthy process for a blind child. It will require a great deal of repeated tactile and kinesthetic readings. What appears to be perseverative behavior, then, is likely to be a highly productive, self-driven strategy for learning and the only one open to such a child. To interfere with this system in favor of the appearance of more typical development is to cause not only incomplete knowledge of objects but also potential problems directly with self-generated learning and mastery motivation. Indirectly, the result of discouraging this kind of adaptation, albeit atypical, has unknowable, pervasive effects on future reorganizations (Lee, 1985).

Learning-disabled children are defined by a deficiency in some area(s) in conjunction with strength in others. This disparity in itself constitutes a disorder. Even if all abilities are above average, the fact that information is being taken in at different levels, with different degrees of mastery, places an excess burden on a child's ability to integrate his or her world. Murphy (1974) describes how this becomes a source of vulnerability:

Typical vulnerable children showed some combination of the following: they were first born; they had had pregnancy or birth difficulties; they were colicky babies and were hard to comfort; they showed a labile pattern of autonomic reactivity; *they were accelerated in certain areas and average or behind their age level in other areas of development – thus finding it hard to integrate the range of basic functions; they had zones of high sensitivity (or reactivity to specific stimuli) or of highly ambivalent responsiveness (intensely pleased by one level or degree of stimulation, then displeased by a slightly more intense or different level)* (Murphy, 1974, p. 89; emphasis ours).

A frequent problem for learning-disabled children involves processes that interfere with the learning of reading. By the time a discrepancy has been identified, most learning-disabled children will have made attempts at deriving effective strategies for circumventing their weaknesses to cope with the demands of reading. When auditory memory weakness underlies the reading problem, children attempt to recognize whole words based on configuration rather than systematic analysis of each letter. Once having achieved some initial sight words, the learning-disabled child is likely to call upon experience as a way to utilize context to discover further words and ultimately meaning. This is a workable strategy for comprehending some passages. In some cases it is also effective in making both child and teacher believe that the child is reading. Nevertheless, the strategy fails to bring such a child to a more explicit understanding of decoding. In fact, it is counterproductive since the entire approach is predicated around the effort to avoid attacking each word systematically. Even when a word is ultimately called correctly, careful observation is likely to establish that the child has never really looked at the components of the word he or she has "read." The strategy is compensatory in that it achieves the goal of normative, adaptive behavior. The child seems comparable to grade placement peers and can perform similarly to them on most worksheets. It is counterproductive in that it fails to lead to true reading skill and must result in failure at levels where the child does not already know about the content and vocabulary.

Counterproductive strategies add a new dimension to the application of typical developmental progressions; when counterproductive strategies exist, "good instruction" (Blankenship, 1978) is likely to meet some opposition. Effective instruction will need to consider those strategies that are natural to the learning-disabled child, who has created them to work within the larger organization of his or her cognitive system. They have brought the child some feeling of success. They might even have been brought to a level of automaticity. It is highly unlikely that a child will be able to override all of this when told the "right" way to do it.

Furthermore, apparently counterproductive or maladaptive behaviors might be a by-product of an organizational system that has evolved to compensate for a more profound, perhaps less obvious disorder. A child with attention deficit and hyperactivity disorder (ADHD) is likely to be impulsive or at least restless; to have difficulty remembering and therefore complying with rules or requests; and to have problems with auditory memory. It is possible, perhaps common, to treat each of these problems individually. Each maladaptive behavior such as blurting one's thoughts aloud, excessive movement, or failure to remember rules might be targeted in a behavior modification program. The auditory memory problem might be treated in the resource room, adaptations in reading instruction might be devised, and modifications in mainstream instruction might be recommended. It is possible, however, that behavior such as speaking aloud is positively driven in the ADHD child. A child with attention and short-term memory problems would do well to try to externalize stimuli rather than to cope with them internally and, thus, place demands on auditory short-term or working memory. Speaking aloud might be less a manifestation of impulsivity than an attempt to transform an auditory memory task into one that is more concrete or "out there." Vygotsky (1962) describes this as typical behavior both developmentally and in adulthood when one is faced with a complex problem. Internal language becomes external as an attempt to make the problem more concrete.

A program for this child will need to consider the chain of effects if negative feedback is given for such behavior. Such an approach would not only jeopardize an effective coping mechanism, but run the risk of upsetting the balance among all the disorders that were at least hypothetically held at bay until now. There is the additional risk of discouraging the child's motivation to evolve compensatory strategies. Certainly talking aloud behavior has the potential for disrupting any classroom, particularly at the young elementary level. A solution that allows the child his or her pattern of coping and the class its own organization might be as simple as teaching or reminding the child to whisper.

We start, then, with the premise that there are qualitative differences that define children with learning disorders. These differences neither exist in isolation nor disappear when a higher-level achievement incorporates them. In the remaining chapters, we attempt to examine issues of differential organization and reorganization within atypical populations.

2
To Err is Human, to Reorganize Divine

A margin of [error] for a maximum of creativity.
                    Revised notes from *The Meet/Meat Room*, J.F. Cawley

Very few systems can operate without error. Even a system that has existed for some time and has operated with a high degree of effectiveness is likely to include some error production. In such a system errors could be a result of a simple mismatch of situation and response; that is, the system attempts to subject a situation to its mode of processing or analysis even though the information is not suitable. Mismatches of this kind can be an accident that allows the system to work effectively in successive instances. Alternately, they can reflect a change in the internal or external environment in which the system operates that requires a reorganization in order for that system to become operative again.

The act of reorganizing is error prone in itself. It is unlikely that a flawless reorganization could evolve at the first stage. In our opinion, it may also be undesirable. Errors made in the early stages of initial organization or reorganization have the potential to serve as units of analysis at later stages of operation. Wallace (1982) refers to the reorganization of a small bank into a larger decentralized banking system as a metaphor for error incidence in a changing cognitive system. Initially, the bank is a small independent enterprise that serves few people, but does so efficiently. Perhaps this bank becomes computerized. After working out the initial bugs in managing the software, the bank evolves into a still more efficient operation. As it becomes more efficient, it is able to offer a greater number of services and to serve a larger population. Greater demands, however, are likely to result, at least initially, in less efficient delivery of services. Perhaps the bank will need to reorganize, decentralize, in order to streamline its operation. The process of decentralization is itself a new one that is likely to be associated with mishaps. Each mishap or error provides feedback for advancement and refinement of the larger system. Once these kinks are worked out, however, the hope is that the bank will operate at maximal efficiency.

In typical cognitive development, information processing systems are in a constant state of reorganization. This reorganization has been viewed in several ways. Stage theories are the most literal representation, where internal schemata are qualitatively ever changing as a result of maturation and interaction with the world. At a more microscopic level, the process of concept formation or strategy generation at any stage can be viewed as a self-modifying system responsive to new information and the desire to operate at the most efficient level.

Regardless of which perspective one assumes, one motivation for reorganization must be related either directly or indirectly to error production or negative feedback. Piaget (1980) and Wason (1972) are explicit about the role of contradiction, conflict, or disequilibrium in the instigation of the refinement of a concept or rule as well as reorganization from a more basic level of operating on information to a higher level one. The typical scenario is that a child or adult learns something, perhaps an arithmetic algorithm, to some level of efficiency and then begins to apply this concept to apparently appropriate events. This approach continues until feedback indicates that the application is not appropriate in a given instance. It is possible, for example, that a child who is beginning to learn how to add is given a pair of two-digit numbers to add that do not require renaming:

$$\begin{array}{r} 13 \\ + \ 12 \\ \hline \end{array}$$

The child might proceed from left to right, figure that $1 + 1 = 2, 3 + 2 = 5$, and arrive at the correct solution. Most children would be given a great deal of experience with items such as these before moving onto the more challenging task of renaming. As a result, it is likely that the child will be quite confident in applying the algorithm when first confronted with a problem such as:

$$\begin{array}{r} 28 \\ + \ 36 \\ \hline \end{array}$$

The solution, 514, will be incorrect. If the child has a real understanding of numbers and is actively monitoring his or her work, the impossibility of this answer might be recognized and result in attempts at reorganization or a request for help. If not, an attentive teacher will recognize the need to point out the error and the need for creating a new algorithm and what that is. Furthermore, the correction device, in the latter case the teacher, will have had some insight into the process that generated the error, which was not available until the error was made. Such an error-correction device makes a certain amount of intuitive sense. Errors are a result of a mismatch between strategy and task demand. But what about those situations in which a child moves from a correct, appropriate, and effective form to an erroneous one? Examples of these are found easily in the literature on language development. Children who were using irregular forms of the past tense such as "went" are likely to switch to "goed" for some period of time and then back to the preferred form (Bowerman, 1982). Children who have mastered the usage of "I" and "Me" are likely to shift temporarily to a stage where some confusion exists (Karmiloff-Smith & Inhelder, 1974/75). These shifts from correct to incorrect are not likely to be a result of environmental disapproval for correct forms. Instead, they seem to be a result of self-initiated efforts at clarifying or analyzing concepts or rule systems. More about both kinds of error production will be said later.

Error occurrence in typical cognitive development, then, is not only inevitable but is associated with stage advancement and concept or strategy refinement. Error production in atypical populations has received a different kind of press. A popular philosophy of teaching children with cognitive disorders advocates error-free learning and guaranteed success. These presumably encourage confidence and a stronger sense of self, and avoid the pitfalls of incorporating misconceptions or faulty strategies into the long-term memory store. We shall argue that error-free learning is in the first place probably not learning at all; that it is not effective in leading to the ultimate goal of establishing what has been variously called frustration tolerance (Murphy, 1974), mastery motivation (Yarrow, Rubenstein, & Pederson, 1975), heartiness in the face of challenge (Dweck, 1987), or ego resiliency (Arend, Gove, & Sroufe, 1979); and that it is a necessary part in the creation of an ever-reorganizing store of knowledge that allows for increasingly greater complexity, integration, and transfer.

Error Production as an Outcome of Data Reduction

Errors are frequently made in all learning endeavors. Even competent learners make errors. Adult learners as well as children are error prone. In fact, people seldom think with the precision attributed to them due to their membership in a particular stage of development (Ennis, 1976; Kohlberg, 1958; Roberge, 1971; Taplin, 1971). This is particularly true when Piaget's rules of formal logic are applied as the standard for correct thinking. Neither adults (Johnson-Laird, 1985; Wason, 1972) nor children (Forman & Cazden, 1985) think typically in precise logical ways. At all ages people tend to avoid acknowledging contradictions or better, alternative solutions. They prefer to assume symmetric relationships, and they prefer to deal with already integrated units of thought at the expense of analyzing component parts. What all of these have in common is their ability to compress, systematize, or reduce information load, albeit at the expense of a valid and complete representation of an experience.

Studies of logic establish the prevalence of errors in adult thinking. Adult thinkers have difficulty when they must decide what is excluded by a proposition. For example, they are likely not to recognize that, given the proposition *if p then q*, when q is the case, that p might or might not be present (Roberge, 1971; Taplin, 1971; Taplin & Staudenmeyer, 1973; Wason & Johnson-Laird, 1972b.) Furthermore, the rule of exclusive disjunction ("or") is the most difficult rule for adults or children to master (Bourne & O'Banion, 1971; Neimark & Slotnick, 1970). The disjunctive rule requires the exclusion of information to form valid inferences.* Wason (1972) makes a point related to this concern about dealing with

---

*The disjunctive "or" requires that one of two propositions connected by it must be true, but not both. In the statement "Mary is married or she is successful," if it is true that Mary is married, the remaining proposition must be negated. Mary is, therefore, not successful.

excluded information. He contends that it is typical to attempt to verify an hypothesis rather than to attempt to find counterevidence. He further describes this "strong obsessional trend" to defend the initial hypothesis as a tendency to view disconfirming evidence as irrelevant.

Perhaps the "obsession" about which Wason remarks is less a tendency to promote one's preferred view or theory and more a tendency to avoid the cognitive demands of considering alternative explanations. The search for exclusions or exceptions has the potential to be infinite. If an exception is not found relatively quickly, the amount of information in working memory becomes increasingly burdensome (Johnson-Laird, 1985). Defense, then, might take the form of avoiding cognitive overload and sheer confusion rather than defense of one's position per se.

Just as exclusion of information is a difficult process for adults and inclusion or generalization is their preference, so are inclusion and generalization typical of the earliest stages of child reasoning. Leopold (1949) reports the tendency to abstract information and to apply it to a large number of instances at the earliest level of semantic development. Brown (1958) alludes to a similar tendency in his description of overgeneralization in the language of children as young as 18 months old. This tendency to generalize, or even to overgeneralize, takes the form of class inclusion in Piaget and Inhelder's (1969) view. From any perspective, it appears that children at a very early age have the ability and propensity to include a wide range of instances into a given set of information. Bower (1964) and Fantz (1961) report instances of such generalization in visual perception of shape and distance in infants as young as 2 months old. By contrast, forms of reasoning that do not allow for simple inclusion are most difficult for children to master. These include valid inferences to be made from conditional and disjunctive statements (Bourne & O'Banion, 1971).

A child's preference for inclusion is not dissimilar from his or her ease at early developmental levels with rules involving symmetrical relationships. The rule of conjunction is the first "formal" logical rule to be mastered by children (Neisser & Weene, 1962). Flavell (1963) describes this early ability as the making of connections, of juxtaposing elements, of judging simply that things go together. Knifong (1974) and Paris (1973) report a similar tendency. Shapiro and O'Brien (1970) call it *child logic* to view conditional statements of the if-then form as if they meant if-and-only-if. This reduces inferences to a series of symmetrical go-together relationships. It is not that children cannot appreciate asymmetrical relationships (Smith, 1979), but rather that the latter requires thinking that is more prone to error.

In both children and adults, then, there is a body of errors that seems to be a result of attempts at data reduction. Since capacity limitations in children are

---

If a negative modifier is included in the negated proposition, processing is that much harder. For example:

John has written his dissertation or he has no job.

If John has written his dissertation, the conclusion is that John has a job.

greater (Case, 1978; Pascual-Leone, 1976), overgeneralization, symmetry, and failure to exclude information are more frequent and more blatant in child than in adult performance. This should not be interpreted, however, as evidence of less or lower-level cognitive activity. The effort to reduce information is in itself an active and effective strategy for understanding that has been described as clustering, chunking, or grouping under laboratory conditions and as script or schema (Nelson, 1987) or frame (Kaye, 1982b) construction in more naturalistic settings. Since it is impossible for the limited-capacity cognitive system to take in all features of an event or situation, some organizing and feature selection is necessary. No understanding can be complete or error free.

Learning-disabled and mildly delayed learners often are defined by their difficulties in coping with larger amounts of information. Traditionally, this difficulty has been attributed to faulty short-term memory (Cherkes-Julkowski, Gertner, & Norlander, 1986). Handicapped learners have been described as lacking organizational strategies that create the format or scheme for chunking or reducing data (Spitz, 1966; Swanson, 1987). More recently, failure to manage large amounts of information has implicated the lack of automatic and efficient processing due to either a neurological weakness or inadequacies in previous learning (Case, 1985; Schiffrin & Dumais, 1981). Ironically, handicapped learners might be less prone to errors of organization than the nonhandicapped. As a result, however, they would be excluded from self-initiated and self-sustained reorganization as well.

Error Production as Evidence of Cognitive Competence

In some sense, then, error production is a result of frame, rule, or strategy generation designed to garner some if not all meaning from an event. It is similar to hypothesis formation. Once having formed a workable frame that explains some if not all aspects of an event and holds some if not all valid implications for other events, it is possible to utilize this frame as a "prototypical episode" (Hundeide, 1985) against which to reference future events. As the frame is applied under additional and varying circumstances, the relationship between it and relevant events becomes more clearly identified. At the same time, each application carries with it a new set of slightly different factors that is fed back and enriches or otherwise modifies the frame. In this way the assimilation–accommodation process (Piaget & Inhelder, 1969) or the dialectic upon which Vygotsky (1981) draws is enacted.

When a frame is evoked, a whole set of tacit correlates are evoked with it. In an efficient system, this happens in an automatic way that detracts little from available capacity. As rich and efficient as this process can be, it produces errors in the form of false expectations and failure to differentiate the details of one event from the stored, prototypical one. Nevertheless, in a restatement of Karmiloff-Smith and Inhelder's (1974/75) theme, you cannot get ahead without a theory, however imperfect.

Assume a stable but multifaceted situtation, such as the presentation of a complex problem of the kind on the Raven Standard Progressive Matrices (Raven, 1958), to be solved in an isolated, uninterrupted setting. One first attempts to frame the information according to some reasonable theory about how the data fit together. If one has been confronted with similar problems, it is likely that some frame is more or less immediately available. Once the frame in constructed, it absorbs problem information relevant to it. The frame itself, whether "correct" or not, serves the very real function of releasing the capacity for examination of further aspects of the problem. In this example, problem solving becomes the dynamic interaction between frame formation-data collection-frame modification-data collection, ad infinitum. The return to data collection serves as a kind of frame-testing or monitoring device. Perhaps the first theory about the Raven puzzle posited that figures progressed systematically, adding additional features each time. Eventually, a figure that fails to conform to this progression is noticed. The contrast between it and the previous theory becomes a prompt for monitoring the original thesis and modifying it. It should not be understood from this example that frames need consist of explicitly stated rules and attributes. Frames, as they are conceptualized in this context, include images and unanalyzed formulations as well. Which kind of frame is actually formulated depends partially on individual differences and partially on task demands. More is said about this in Chapter 3.

Error production in this context signals the learner/solver that a reformulation of one's perspective is necessary and also reveals at a more explicit level to the teacher, to the diagnostician, or to the solver what the previous theory was and what it allowed and disallowed. They are "good" errors in that they are evidence of frame formulation. They are "lawful" to the extent that they are applications of otherwise viable principles. The typical example here is the overextension of the past tense inflection by young children ("daddy goed"). Likewise, lawful errors might include the previous example of adding from left to right. Children who have overextended this algorithm have done so because they have constructed a rule and found it to be effective in all of their experiences thus far.

The act of making an error is a virtue in itself. It indicates that some self-generated processing is taking place. After all, the child who says "daddy goed" or who adds 28 + 36 to produce 514 has not been told by others to do this. In both instances, the child has decided upon a likely strategy and has decided to use it. Without this underlying activity no future, more effective strategies can be generated. Furthermore, if these errors occur with any regularity, they reveal the way a child thinks. Armed with this information, teachers can be quite effective in deciding how to proceed with instruction. Without it, they will be able to make only blind attempts at altering the child's approach to learning, or worse, will attempt merely to modify a response.

All three of these examples, the Raven task, expressive language development, and the formation of arithmetic algorithms, have been topics for examining learning disorders and delays. The impaired learner is characterized as relatively rigid in his or her efforts. In algorithm application, Brown (1978) refers to this as blind rule following. In the Raven task the learner is described as lacking focused attention or as passive (Budoff & Corman, 1976). In communication situations the learner is likely not to detect when a communication attempt has failed (Donahue, 1986). Observations of learning-disabled students attempting to solve the Raven patterns are enlightening. Typically, they begin quite well, even with the more abstract problems having fewer lines and configurations. When asked to verbalize their reasons for selecting correct choices, they are often very vague. Nevertheless, they remain confident in their decision. This lack of explicit awareness of what the problem is as well as the procedure for solution seems to be more than an isolated difficulty with expressive language. Many of these children are quite competent with linguistic expression under other conditions. Their nonhandicapped peers tend to begin at an implicit level as well. Nonhandicapped solvers, however, tend to confront their confusions and their errors more boldly and to drive their understanding of the problems to a more explicit level where it can be modified. It is at this point that many learning-disabled youngsters will simply quit. If urged to try, they will respond by impulsively finishing each pattern in the time it takes to turn the page and move one's finger. The only intervention that has appeared to be effective is to decompose the problem by pointing systematically and gradually to each of its components (Budoff & Corman, 1976). Learning-disabled youngsters, then, seem to reach a point where they simply defend against input, input from the problem directly as well as input in the form of feedback about their initial attempts. Such a defense is reminiscent of the self-protection against overload to which Johnson-Laird (1985) refers.

Error Detection and Correction

The ability to formulate an initial, albeit very possibly erroneous strategy, then, is an important component of competent learning. Error commission is effective in the process of self-instruction, however, only to the extent that there is a self-correction device. If no self-monitoring takes place, if errors are made and simply ignored (DeLoache, Sugarman, & Brown, 1981; Wason, 1972) to the extent that they have not become habitual, they serve neither a productive nor a counterproductive purpose in information acquisition or understanding. The more abstract the operation, the less likely that errors will be detected. Unless our arithmetic student understands the value of three-digit numbers, the impossibility of the sum 514 is not likely to be recognized. Piaget and Inhelder (1969), among others (Feuerstein, Jensen, Hoffman, & Rand, 1985), have made a point of the value of direct, concrete experience. What might be the virtue of concrete manipulation is not its cognitive simplicity, but the necessity of acknowledging wrong moves. When a larger nesting cup does not slip into a smaller one, it is difficult to ignore this feedback. Even very young children (1 to 1½ years old) will recognize that they are at an impasse (DeLoache et al., 1981). They may not be able to derive an effective strategy, but they give evidence of recognizing the mismatch in the form of examining the nonnesting cup as if to discover what has gone wrong with it.

When direct, material feedback is not available, it often becomes the role of an informed adult to mediate (Feuerstein et al., 1985) or regulate the experience (Kaye, 1982a, 1982b). A child who calls a tiger a kitty might be told that it is a very big cat indeed and is called a tiger. In this way, the child recognizes that the frame or category for cat needs some modifications. The mediator need not always be an adult. There is a popular truism that many children are handicapped only from 9 to 3. During their nonacademic day, they are "street wise." Facility with everyday cognitions might, in part, be due to their interpersonal nature. Children or adults operating in groups are likely to be reminded, either gently or not so gently, that they are in error and to be confronted with conflicting information (Cherkes-Julkowski et al., 1986). The role of social groups in cognition is discussed in more detail in Chapter 5.

Eventually, regardless of the availability of direct or mediated feedback, a competent learner takes on the self-regulatory, metaoperational function of judging whether an error has been committed. Learning-disabled children, on the other hand, do not seem to be able to assume this role with any ease. The metacognitive literature points out repeatedly that learning-disabled and mentally retarded children fail to evaluate whether their approach is leading in the right direction or whether their performance has been adequate (Brown, Bransford, Ferrara, & Campione, 1983).

Effective feedback about errors need not provide a correct solution. The most basic and earliest form of feedback is the kind of direct, material feedback exemplified by DeLoache and co-workers' (1981) toddlers, who recognized that the larger cup would not fit in the smaller one. There is some suggestion that the most valuable form of feedback is that which results from self-initiated attempts that activate approaches to structuring the problem and then draw attention to the failure of an individual's strategy or frame (Kaye, 1982b). Under conditions of self-initiation of this kind, feedback about errors reactivates the child's frame formation or frame application system. In contrast, feedback that provides a whole solution deactivates these processes. In the first case the child must construct a solution based on personal perspective rather than adopt the perspective of the other. The advantages are somewhat greater than what is implied simply by discovery learning. The creation of the new solution is a gain in its own right and serves to build a new frame upon which to build other strategies. In addition, the old strategy, which was erroneously applied, becomes modified. Its limitations are more evident. If more than one strategy has been attempted prior to solution, all of these have been refined to some degree. For handicapped learners, the advantages of feedback that indicates an error has been made and does not attempt to impose "corrective" approaches are even more significant. Almost all handicaps to learning involve disorders of attention, including the selection of critical features (Zeaman & House, 1979) capacity for processing information in working memory (Case, 1985; Spitz, 1966), and adequate deployment of attention (Krakow & Kopp, 1983). Once actively involved in the problem solving/

learning process, the child has already decided upon a focus and perspective. To ask this child to adopt the perspective of an "expert" makes cognitive/attentional demands that are simply too great (Rocissano & Yatchmink, 1983).

If one accepts that frames do not exist in isolation, each modification of an existing frame or addition of a new frame modifies the entire organization of the transactional system (Kaye, 1982b; Sameroff, 1982). The end result of error feedback, then, is that the network of strategies or frames evoked and modified is adjusted and embellished to include more intricate connections. Even if the problem is not solved, the opportunity for higher-level reorganization of or within the larger system is a valuable component of error commission and detection.

"Error-Free" Learning and Passivity

There are children who are discouraged from making errors, either due to their own beliefs about success and failure (Weiner, 1974) or what intelligence and success are (Dweck, 1987) or due to environments that "protect" them from going astray. Indeed these two factors, internal (self-attributions) and external (environmental), can hardly be considered as independent. Failure to commit errors is a syndrome reflective of a complex of disorders. Since nothing can be learned with full appreciation for complexity and richness without efforts at actively formulating, testing, and refining one's frame, avoidance of errors must mean avoidance of active processing and ultimately of active strategic behavior. Without feedback from erroneous attempts, meaningful hierarchical reorganization is difficult to envision. Typically, either as antecedent or consequent, children who are error avoidant are part of an interactional system between self and parent in the early years and between self and school personnel later in which the adult brings the world to the child prepackaged and already processed. The cycle continues to produce increasing passivity (Stern & Hildebrandt, 1986) and thus an increasing need to deliver information to the child in a fashion that requires the least active involvement on the child's part. This pattern of continuous, guaranteed "success" results in behaviors and attitudes associated with passivity and allowing others to structure information and procedures. Such a continuous reinforcement schedule produces behaviors that are easily extinguished according to a behavioral model. In explanations for success and failure according to an attribution model, the result is external attributions and an external locus of control that is inversely associated with mastery motivation. Both models emphasize the value of trials or attempts that are not reinforced/successful in establishing frustration tolerance and the association of initial difficulty with ultimate success.

Many of the children who end up identified as passive learners (Torgesen, 1980; Wong, 1980) with low frustration tolerance and external attributions about success and failure are those who were vulnerable either at birth or during the initial stages of development. For many of these children, a cycle in which adults initiate and establish the focus of attention as well as the topic of "conversation" begins during the first days of life. Preterm infants have been identified as the prototype of children at risk for handicaps (Parmalee, 1981). Prematurity embodies the potential for nearly all risk factors that constitute early vulnerability: health and neurological impairment, nutritional deprivation during the pre- and postnatal periods, teenage pregnancy and mothering styles, and stresses due to poverty, family situation, or other emotional factors. The incidence of retardation and learning disorders is higher in preterm infants than in the general population. Much of the study of child passivity comes from work done with this population. Another large portion of the early development literature includes studies of children with Down's syndrome, since it is a form of actual learning impairment identifiable, except in rare instances, at birth.

Preterm infants are described as having difficulty in maintaining and thus signaling their state and in general cuing their caregivers as to their wants and needs (Goldberg & DeVitto, 1983). In the absence of clear communications about hunger, discomfort, and desire for interaction/stimulation, the caretaker is left with the responsibility of deciding when and how the child should be fed, stimulated, and so on. Ironically, this has often resulted in a pattern in which parents tend to provide an amount of stimulation the infant cannot tolerate at an inappropriate time. The result is an irritable, unresponsive child or, in the case of a better-organized infant, one who is able to avert to prevent overstimulation. If this pattern is allowed to establish itself, one can well imagine the contribution it makes to reduced active and initiating processing as well as to disorders in communication.

Preterm infants and those with Down's syndrome tend to initiate less (Field, 1977; Jones, 1980) and to have longer response latencies than nonrisk infants. Some of this tendency seems to be a result of reduced alertness due to problems in state regulation and to general disorganization of the central nervous system (Thoman, 1987). Nevertheless, a question remains concerning the degree to which the condition is exacerbated by the child-caretaker system. In the absence of initiations by the child, concerned parents are likely to draw their child's attention to things, demonstrate toy play, and direct the child's interactions with the social and inanimate world. Parent-directed interactions of this kind present a greater cognitive and state-regulating demand on the child. The demand is made on the child to discern and then adapt to the adult's focus of attention. This is a nearly impossible act for a novice to accomplish beyond the chance level (Rocissano & Yatchmink, 1983). Beyond this, it exhausts a young child's cognitive capacity, resulting in no remaining capacity for the intake and processing of the information that was the original topic of interaction (Schiffrin & Dumais, 1981). If the demands are too great, the end result will be to disorganize the child completely and create not only a failed episode but a general aversion to this kind of arousal. Sameroff and Chandler (1975) refer to this dynamic as the "continuum of caretaking casualty."

In addition, parents of infants at risk are exposed to the very early and very real vulnerability of their children. In the case of preterm infants and some children with Down's syndrome, health problems are enormous. As infants they tend to be physically weaker and less stable. A sense of protectiveness, perhaps overprotectiveness, is established at birth (Stern & Hildebrandt, 1986). This stereotype of the preterm infant seems to persist well beyond the stage at which the infants have gained age-appropriate levels of development (Barnard, Bee, & Hammond, 1984; Stern & Hildebrandt, 1986; Cherkes-Julkowski, Bertrand, Roth, & Bradley, 1987). The stereotype of the child as passive and in need of external direction seems to persist during the preschool years and is adopted by the special education system upon school entry.

We have pursued the investigation of mother's teaching styles with preterm and full-term children as part of a larger longitudinal study (Cherkes-Julkowski et al., 1987). When their children are 20 months old (for preterm infants, 20 months from expected date of birth), mothers of preterm infants are far more directive than mothers of full-term children. They tend to structure the environment, to establish their focal point and their topic, and to physically prompt their children into acceptable responses. Degree of directiveness effectively discriminates between preterm and full-term dyads. The interesting aspect of these data is that degree of directiveness is *not* related to any particular characteristic of the child. Developmental levels at 5 and 13 months, as measured by the Dunst (1980) revision of Uzgiris and Hunt's Ordinal Scales of Psychological Development (1975) at 5 and 13 months, fail to predict maternal directiveness at 20 months. Likewise, neither Socioeconomic Status (SES) nor the child's level of psychosocial development at 5 and 13 months, as measured by Foley and Hobin's Attachment-Separation-Individuation Scale (1981), is predictive. The only factors that yield more than the most modest of relationships are measures of maternal responsiveness at early ages (0.7) and degree of initial prematurity (0.75). There appears to be a style of mothering that persists at least from 5 months forward that fails to recognize the identity and the personal style of the child and instead imposes an organization on the child's world according to some standard that seems appropriate for optimizing development. Since the children are not very different in actual developmental age, mothers must be responding to something else. Perhaps there are qualitative behavioral differences in our two groups of children to which our measures are not sensitive. We pursued this idea as we watched videotapes of children playing. Trained observers naive to the classification of preterm versus full term were not able to identify with any certainty which child belonged to which category. Mothers seem to be reacting to some stereotype of vulnerability and diminished competence directly related to the degree of initial prematurity.

Maternal estimates of children's competence have been found to be related to mothers' verbal interactional styles with their children. Mervis (1984) reports an intriguing comparison of full-term and preterm mothers' approaches to language instruction. Mothers of full-term infants tend to adapt to the focus of their children, to recognize what is salient to them, and to accept their children's view. For example, a round candle or a round bank is likely to be called a ball by an 18-month-old who is beginning to learn language. Mothers of full-term children accept these "errors" without correction. It is only when the child begins to attend to those features that are critical aspects of the object's identity in another, more conventional class (the wick or the slot for coins) that mothers of full-term children suggest that this object is actually not a ball but a candle or a bank. They allow a great deal of practice in extending the concept of ball. In addition, they seem to wait until the child has noticed enough information about objects so that self-detection of the "error" is possible. It is at that point that the full-term mother feeds back to the child that this one is, for example, a candle. Preterm mothers are quite different. They are always on the alert to provide the correct label regardless of the child's basis for organizing the world. Interestingly, Cardoso-Martins, Mervis, and Mervis (1985) provide some indirect evidence that maternal teaching styles of this kind depress vocabulary development below that which might be expected from developmental age and delay.

It is difficult to predict exactly what the effects of early protection from self-initiated play and interactions might be. Stern and Hildebrandt (1986) have established the existence of a preterm stereotype in their study of adult play with full-term infants, half of whom were, for experimental purposes, misleadingly identified as preterm. They were able to uncover a reliable trend for play with preterm children that consisted of the attitude that such children are more fragile, less likable, and less approachable than full-term children. In addition, there is no evidence that this attitude resolves itself as preterm children become better organized and developmentally equivalent to their full-term peers (Barnard et al., 1984; Stern & Hildebrandt, 1986). At 2 years, however, preterm infants, regardless of their developmental status, seem to be more passive and diffuse in play and in interpersonal interaction (Cherkes-Julkowski et al., 1987). Whether this passivity is a result of initial biological insult, environmental interference, or some interaction between these factors is not yet known. Nevertheless, the early establishment of a passive learning style and the stereotyped expectation on the part of parents that their child's investigations must be orchestrated and engineered into an "acceptable" outcome cannot be without effect on one's approach to learning, at least in the preschool and early school years.

Not the least of the effects of early passivity must be its contribution to the determination of self, curiosity, and resiliency in the face of problem solving. These, in turn, affect motivational style (Arend et al., 1979; Weiner, 1974). Dweck (1987) has established two groups of school-age children with distinctly different motivational styles. These are the familiar ones: those children who retreat at initial defeat and those who become "hearty" in the face of a challenge. She suggests that motivational styles are mediated by a child's belief about the nature of intelligence. If they have come to understand that intelligence is a fixed and steady trait, they tend to focus on immediate, error-free success as testimony to their ability. Others have a view of a more dynamic, incremental intelligence. Those with this view believe that when they are learning they are enhancing their abilities. Typical styles of interacting with very young, vulnerable, and handicapped children suggest in subtle and not-so-subtle ways that correct performance, particularly performance without error, is pleasing to adults and, therefore, must be the desired way of learning. Furthermore, the expectation is that adults prefer to structure the entire episode so that the most "intelligent" outcome will be facilitated. One manifestation of this is the use of developmental checklists such as the Learning Accomplishment Profile (Stanford, 1978) or criterion-referenced tests as a basis for intervention. The goal is to steer the child on an upward course through the continuum as quickly as possible. Errors or regressions are taken as evidence of inability in the child or deficiency in instruction.

Typical instructional techniques with handicapped students do much to promote this expectation. Instruction tends to value error-free learning and guaranteed success. The approach is justified by its goal of increasing self-confidence and self-worth as well as its ability to ensure accurate performance. Neither can be accepted as accurate. Ego resiliency (Arend et al., 1979), internal attribution to one's cognitive ability (Weiner, 1974), or mastery motivation (Yarrow et al., 1975) are associated with endurance in the face of false starts. Problem solving involves effortful and multiple attempts in the face of an unknown entity. The need to do some figuring and to design alternative strategies defines the problem situation. Without the expectation that solutions are often accompanied, indeed predicted (Amsel & Roussel, 1952), by initial failure, there is not problem solving. Effective teaching has somehow become associated with the guarantee of immediately successful outcomes rather than the encouragement of independence as a problem solver, albeit one who must commit errors and suffer false starts. "Effective" teaching would consist of imparting correct solutions to children, preferably in one step. It would be less concerned with guiding a child in self-analysis of error-prone attempts at solution. Ironically, preschool teachers are less effective at helping preschool children to modify their messages in referential communication tasks than either mothers or adults who have neither their own children nor experience working with the children of others (Bertrand, 1987).

Optimally, error production becomes associated with the path to success and takes on a quality of anticipatory goal response (Amsel & Roussel, 1952). In addition, in an active processing system, each error feeds back to the initial conceptualization of the problem and the strategies designed for its solution. Hall and Day (1982) provide evidence that in learning-disabled children a greater number of errors during initial learning is associated with improved transfer. Our own work in strategy training indicates a similar trend. A greater number of errors during initial training correlates with success on a posttest task (Cherkes-Julkowski et al., 1986).

For errors to be motivating or at least tolerated, they must be associated positively with a range of task-related events. One of these is a sense of success or goal attainment. Another is the accepting and encouraging attitude of the teacher or other who is guiding the learner. A child who is meeting difficulty in an atmosphere where errors are condemned or even just allowed is not likely to see mistakes as motivating. Where errors are received positively, perhaps with humor and the encouraging feedback that one has learned yet another bit of useful information, they have a rich potential for personal and cognitive growth.

Error Commission and Regression

It is tempting to assume a rather direct and linear relationship between the frequency and kind of error commission on the one hand and the competence and sophistication of the learner on the other. Younger and less experienced adults or children would be expected to make a greater number of errors than those who are developmentally more advanced or better initiated. There is, however, some evidence for a U-shaped learning curve (Karmiloff-Smith & Inhelder, 1974/75; Strauss, 1982; Thelen, 1986), which describes initial success, a drop in performance, and finally an advance to a more highly competent level.

The U-shaped curve has been found across broad stages as well as at a more microscopic level of skill acquisition. Evidence of conservation of number (Strauss & Curtis, 1984) has been found as early as 10 months of age and at the ages of 3 and 4 years. Nevertheless, at approximately 5 years of age children begin making errors on the conservation task, only to perform accurately again during the early elementary years (Piaget & Inhelder, 1969). Similar evidence has been found for conservation of weight in the second year of life (Monoud & Bower, 1975), with a decline and apparent reemergence at the age of 8 years. At a microscopic level children have been observed to generate solutions to a problem that are correct but that tend to be rather more cumbersome and piecemeal than desired (Karmiloff-Smith, 1979). There seems to be a drive toward improved, more efficient and sophisticated strategies. Nevertheless, the progress from initial success to a later, higher level of success requires a reorganization of cognitive processes. Error commission and detection are something more than accidents resulting from environmental feedback and, it is hoped, self-correction. Errors of these kind reflect an internally driven reorganization process that seeks a higher-level structure.

There are a series of explanations about what the nature of this reorganization might be (Strauss, 1982). It is possible that something new is learned first at an implicit or unanalyzed level. Eventually, seemingly as a result of a drive toward improved and more parsimonious explanations (Bowerman, 1982; Karmiloff-Smith, 1979), the learner attempts to derive an explicit rule that would have the advantage of explaining the present set of data, of reducing information load by abstracting the most critical features, and possibly of being generalizable to future situations. So, the novice is likely to adopt workable although low-level principles. In an effort to find an underlying universal principle, however, the novice is likely to construct an explicit rule and to be less receptive to exceptions or special cases. At this stage, a young child might overextend the "-ed" ending for past tense verbs or may attempt to borrow in all places of a subtraction problem whether indicated or not. In this way the U-shaped curve begins to be constructed. It begins with a relatively high rate of initial, implicit, relatively automatic, but limited "correct" responding. Eventually learners become more aware of the regularities of their responses. They become less automatic in their responses and more mindful of the rule system or strategy itself. In the effort to analyze their rule system they appear less confident and clumsier in their application of previously automatic strategies. Many examples have been offered to illustrate the awkwardness of performing automatic acts at an explicitly conscious level: carrying a full cup of coffee, walking, speaking. Nevertheless, the initial dip in performance during the analysis or reanalysis stage does yield a higher, more abstract, more fully analyzed level of understanding.

The transition from implicit awareness or perhaps an heuristic approach to processing (Howe, Brainerd, & Kingma, 1985) to a more explicit one is not a natural progression for learning-disabled students. Because they are disorganized, passive, lack executive control, or have impaired abilities in achieving an efficient use of capacity, because of learned helplessness, or because of any combination of these, it is not likely that they would make an unprompted shift from initial workable procedures to harder-to-achieve and more cumbersome ones. Unfortunately, looser, unanalyzed procedures do not predict well to the learning of symbol systems in reading or in mathematics. Unanalyzed procedures are not to be panned as entirely or even partially worthless. Some very complex situations require more fluid, less explicit analyses as a way of absorbing the richness of a situation while still defending against overload. Some situations, such as learning in context, allow for a more implicit understanding that accepts unanalyzed frames imposed by repeated experience. Symbol learning, however, requires willful, out-of-context, arbitrary associations (Goodnow, 1976; Olson, 1976). It is at this point in their schooling that many learning-disabled youngsters become identified.

Strauss (1982) suggests that rather than a progression from unanalyzed to analyzed forms, reorganization is driven by a transition from lower-level schemes for knowing to higher-level ones. Knowledge of the relationship between weight and size or number and space might be at a sensory/motor stage at first. When awareness moves to a representational level with an algebraic base, some initial confusion is to be expected. Likewise, a move from a representational to an abstract, formal/symbolic system must cause some initial disarray.

According to any of these explanations, an individual's internal system for organizing information is constantly changing. In an efficient system, each successive reorganization creates a more intricately structured knowledge store, which allows for the greatest amount of information to be stored by preserving the greatest amount of regularity while avoiding as much overlap as possible (Wallace, 1982). The knowledge or long-term memory store has a complex organization of nested subroutines that are triggered in appropriate sequence according to environmental demands (Kaye, 1982a, 1982b). Since no intentional act can be orchestrated without coordinating a number of schemata, the integrity and efficiency of the system at large are of major importance. Growth in the system allows for more complex solutions. Conflict and conflict resolution play a major role in signaling the need for reorganization.

For an error commission-feedback-correction loop to function effectively, a number of components must be in place, most of which are not easily accessed by children with learning disorders. In the first place, the initially organized system must have a structure with enough clarity so that a fault in the system is obvious. If it is too loosely organized, all things are possible within it and mistakes do not give pause or reason for higher-level reorganization. Herein lies a connection between the stereotyped passivity, this time in the face of conflict, and the stereotyped disorganization of the learning disabled.

Furthermore, the orchestration of a multiroutine system is cumbersome. It demands a great deal of prowess in attending to and managing large amounts of information and a number of procedures. This is achieved in the best of circumstances only through increasing automaticity with previously learned subroutines and their coordination. It is this automaticity that allows for limited capacity to be allocated for new learning. Learning-disabled children are notorious for their lack of automaticity (Schiffrin & Dumais, 1981; Swanson, 1987) and their capacity limitations (Swanson, 1987).

Error Production as a Key to Assessment and Instruction

Error commission, then, reflects the level and kind of cognitive organization that learners have at their disposal. To the extent that error is a result of the learners' own attempts and to the extent that they recognize the conflict between their intended goal and the actual outcome, error commission serves as a trigger for improved, higher-level reorganization. Educationally, the error commission-recognition-reorganization device is a powerful one. Its benefits to the efficient learner are self-evident. Since impaired learners typically do not monitor their performance or reevaluate the outcome of their efforts (Brown et al,. 1983) the internal feedback system is less likely to promote meaningful reorganization. Nevertheless, it is possible for an external agent to monitor error production and to be the source of metacognitive reorganization (Belsky, Garduque, & Hrncir, 1984; Feuerstein et al., 1985; Kaye, 1982a, 1982b). It should become, then, a primary emphasis of teachers of children with learning problems to allow their students to make errors and to use them to interpret the internal organization of the learner. It becomes possible to adapt instruction to the child's initial perspective and progress from here to continually higher levels of organization.

In this view, knowing how the child approaches or structures a problem is a critical piece of information in the formulation of individualized instruction. Once cognitive style is identified, it can be used in a series of constructive ways in the selection of instructional strategies. First, if the teacher knows what structures, what frames of reference a child has, it becomes an easier matter to fit a new bit of information into the child's already existing store of information. Ausubel and Fitzgerald (1962) call this *meaningful learning*. For example, if one is trying to teach the concept of fractions and knows that the child has an understanding of parts that make up wholes, here might be the perspective from which to begin. If we want to teach the concept of middle and we know the child understands betweenness, we might begin within this frame. In fact, if a mentally handicapped child has a given procedure for structuring information and if instruction is not compatible with it, the mismatch might seriously endanger the effectiveness of instruction. Second, then, we have to have some concern for whether a child's set of strategies can be used to facilitate learning or must, instead, be avoided. If it is decided that a given strategy is detrimental, the issue becomes whether instruction should resort to a direct introduction of an adequate strategy or whether instruction needs to consider in some way the misleading one. The danger of ignoring the misleading strategy is that the child is used to it. It is likely that the strategy is triggered in an almost automatic way whenever a related problem is presented. In the case of the math example presented on page 19, it is most likely that the child will approach addition computations from left to right. It is not enough that we demonstrate a right-to-left progression. This child, through force of habit if not conviction, will want to go from left to right. Herein might lie one source of the common complaint that a child seems to know it one day but not the next. Indeed, the child can do it the "right" way when reminded of the appropriate algorithm. Left to his or her own devices, however, the child opts for (or is at the mercy of) the old, well-established set of responses. If the decision is to ignore the old strategy and simply train on the "right" one, it is necessary to acknowledge that a great deal of drilling will be necessary. The amount of drilling is determined, at least in part, by the strength of the previous strategy preference. In other words, it is possible that the child would need to practice the new, right way more than he or she has already practiced (maybe for years) the old way. Perhaps a more efficient instructional device would be to show the child how to use the old strategy effectively. In this case, a series of repeated addition might be appropriate:

$$
\begin{array}{r}
28 \\
+\ 36 \\
\hline
50 \\
+\ 14 \\
\hline
64
\end{array}
$$

If a teacher is committed to instructing the child in the traditional algorithm, it becomes necessary to present problems in a way that interferes with the child's tendency to apply the old, inappropriate strategy. In our example, one way would be to provide the answer and to have the child place the carried number in the appropriate position. The problem would look like this:

$$
\begin{array}{r}
3486 \\
+\ 2354 \\
\hline
5840
\end{array}
$$

The child's response would be

$$
\begin{array}{r}
11 \\
3486 \\
+\ 2354 \\
\hline
5840
\end{array}
$$

There is certainly no guarantee that the correct strategy will be used automatically. Nevertheless, by changing the characteristics of the stimulus, it is less likely that the old response set will be triggered.

Error analysis of this kind is justified by the belief that understanding exactly why the child is having difficulty is important in understanding the problem and, thus, in planning the most efficient and effective intervention. The goal in error analysis is to identify the child's conceptual organization and its context rather than simply to delineate each area that has not been mastered. Once the source has been identified and understood in the larger cognitive organization of the learner, instruction can be designed to attack the problem at this most basic level and by so doing to have the potential for the greatest generalization or application in the widest range of circumstances, as well as the potential for meaningful, higher-level reorganization. The alternative to this approach, the delineation of nonmastered areas, leaves room only for separate, discrete instruction in each area. The contention here is that this latter approach to instruction is not only uneconomical but probably discourages rather than encourages understanding, complex reorganization, and meaningful growth of the larger cognitive system.

Take, for example, a child's responses on a mathematics test. Table 2.1 displays a sample performance. This child has made errors in items 3, 9, 10, and 11. One approach would be to plan four sets of lessons including carrying in addition, borrowing in subtraction, writing three-digit numerals, and sequencing three-digit numerals. This plan would involve a continuum of steps in each of these four areas, and each would take a learner of average speed a considerable amount of time. The approach suggested here recommends something quite different. First, the diagnostician is encouraged to explain why the child was able to do items 1, 2, 4, 5, 6, 7, and 8 correctly, but not the others. Clearly, the student knows the facts or can figure them out and can do multiple-column operations with accuracy. The theme that seems to be common to those items on which the child faltered is place value. An examination of the nature of the incorrect responses indicates, again, knowledge of facts, but failure to understand the constraints of place value. In each of the incorrect items, however, the child is attempting to extend the knowledge and procedures that are under his or her command. The

TABLE 2.1. Responses to a series of arithmetic items.

1.	1	2.	6	3.	17	4.	123	5.	9
	+ 3		+ 7		+ 39		+ 241		− 2
	4		13		416		364		5
6.	13	7.	39	8.	687	9.	42		
	− 2		− 22		− 232		− 18		
	11		17		455		36		

10. Write a numeral for "three hundred two": 32

11. Finish this row of numbers:

298, 299, 2910, 2911, 2912

plan for instruction that would result from such an analysis begins with a complete explanation of place value. Perhaps this would include concrete materials, expanded notation, or conversion of numbers to different bases. In any case, the intent would be to treat the faulty concept underlying the mistakes across items. The assumption is that once the concept of place value has been understood, it will be an easy transfer to carrying, borrowing, numeral writing, and sequencing, as well as to advanced multiplication and division.

The actual procedure of error analysis suggested here, then, involves three basic steps: (1) establishing patterns of correct and incorrect responses; (2) delineating the nature of the errors made; and (3) interpreting the underlying cognitive state that could have generated those responses in that particular pattern. The intent in the following section is to demonstrate how each of these steps can be worked and applied to instruction.

Diagnosing Patterns of Correct and Incorrect Responses

Any learning that requires more than the most rigid response to a unique stimulus requires some understanding of the expanse and limitations of the concept of skill involved. So, looking at any one response to any one item in any area can yield only limited information about the extent to which a student has learned a concept. To identify exactly what the child has come to understand and has included as elements in personal rules or categorizations requires observations in a series of related situations. The child's pattern of strengths and weaknesses will define for the diagnostician the extent to which the concept has been understood. The child in Table 2.1, for example, demonstrates some knowledge of number concept, subtraction, place value, and sequencing, but fails to demonstrate full understanding of any of these. If the child understood subtraction thoroughly, he or she would respect the fact that its terms were not commutative and would not, as in item 9, subtract 2 from 8. The child does have some inkling of place value, because the integrity of each column in each of the operations is respected. The child is simply unaware of regrouping within a single number (i.e., 4 tens + 16 ones = 5 tens + 6 ones). Some knowledge of sequencing is evidenced by the fact that only the digit in the far right position of the numeral (item 11) is changed, and this is done correctly. The child fails only to demonstrate an ability to regroup within a single number. It is the *pattern* of right and wrong answers that provides the basis for identifying the nature of an individual child's understanding of a concept or concepts by revealing the interconnection between related concepts or experiences stored in the child's episodic memory (Chi, 1985).

Searching for patterns of strength and weakness is equally important in diagnosing the more general area of cognitive style strengths and weaknesses. Some instruments are designed to evaluate not mastery of specific content, but more general characteristics of learning abilities and styles. The Detroit Tests of Learning Aptitude−2 (Hammill, 1985) is a case in point. Assume for a moment that we can have confidence in Detroit scores, in the norms, and in the comparison

TABLE 2.2. Scores for the two hypothetical children on subtests of the Detroit Tests of Learning Aptitude – 2.

John		Mary	
Word Opposites	14	Symbolic Relations	15
Sentence Imitation	13	Word Opposites	7
Conceptual Matching	14	Object Sequences	14
Word Sequences	8	Word Sequences	12
Object Sequences	7	Conceptual Matching	8

among scores. Assumptions about validity and reliability are less risky in the renormed form. The goal for the diagnostician is then to search for a pattern of strengths and weaknesses that can help to characterize the child as a learner. Consider the two profiles based on Detroit findings presented in Table 2.2. John and Mary are the same chronologic age. They have the same average level of functioning. The question becomes whether they, therefore, possess similar learning propensities. If we can believe patterns of strengths and weaknesses on the Detroit Tests, they do not. However, why would John, for example, perform in just this way? What kind of learner would do well on Word Opposites, Conceptual Matching, and Sentence Imitation? What kind of a learner would experience most difficulty with Object Sequences and Word Sequences? An examination of each of these subtests suggests a pattern. Each of the subtests on which John scored above the mean score provides the child with a set of structured information to which he must respond. In the word opposites and conceptual matching tests, the child is given the relationship (different, similar) and asked to complete the terms or explain them. In the third, Sentence Imitation, the child hears a sentence, has access to fully organized utterances, and must repeat them. The tests that have proved difficult for John, in contrast, provide no structure, no organization for the child and, thus, increase demands on attention and working memory. In the sequencing tests, the child hears or sees separate, disconnected bits of information and is required to find some way to make sense out of nonsense.

Mary is different. Her performance does not divide out on the basis of structured-nonstructured tasks. She does well on one highly structured task, Symbolic Relations, but poorly on other structured tasks, Word Opposites and Conceptual Matching. She also does well on some unstructured tasks, Object and Word Sequences. Her performance does not seem to split along the dimension auditory-visual. Again, the scores are high on some pictorial or visual tasks, but not on others; high on some auditory or verbal tasks, low on others. An examination of the tests suggests that Mary performs best when the task does not require the mastery of previously learned content. On these tests Mary seems able to work with any information given her and to process it effectively. When the task requires knowledge of vocabulary (Word Opposites) or awareness of expected relationships (Conceptual Matching), she seems to lack the background needed.

John, then, appears to need help in the area of approaching information strategically. Without it, he has real difficulty mastering new information. Mary is nearly his opposite. Learning new things presents no difficulty for her. In fact, the newer the better, since what she appears to lack is a store of previously acquired content. The intervention for John should involve both an effort to encourage self-generated attempts at organizing information and techniques for delivering information that he needs in a well-structured way to avoid aggravating his weakest abilities. For Mary, the exact style of instruction does not seem so critical. What does appear to be necessary is the provision of a wide range of experiences upon which she can draw in later learning.

Patterns can be analyzed in a slightly different way. In another hypothetical case, Susan has taken the Gallistel-Ellis Test of Coding Skills. Table 2.3 enumerates some of her correct answers and phonetic spellings of the errors she made. She read "jod" instead of *job*; "hud" instead of *hub*; and "wed" instead of *web*. It is tempting to conclude that she reverses. However, she read *big*, *kid*, and *red* correctly. Also, in the second section, she read *prod* and *slob* correctly. In fact, her correct reading of *b* and *d* occurs more frequently than her incorrect reading. She can tell the difference, and she knows the sound. Again, in Section II, she makes errors in the words *spun*, *smell*, and *ject*. In these she misreads the short *u* sound, which she reads consistently correctly in nine other words. She omits the "s" in the "sm" blend, but blends "s" accurately all of the seven other times. The diagnostician needs to search for the reason Susan makes these errors in these contexts. It could be attributed to insignificant carelessness. A probe consisting of instructions to look at the misread words again and to reread them would provide further information about this possibility. Susan's mistakes could be due to greater confusion when the "b" appears at the end of the word; however, her reading of *clob* and even *prod* discourages this explanation. One could argue that when a word is unfamiliar to Susan she falters in some area, even though she can demonstrate mastery in that same area in a simpler more familiar situation. This explanation is likewise unsupportable, however, since she reads 9 of 10 nonsense words correctly.

No response, then, exists in isolation. In Susan's case, what initially appeared to be an error requiring some attention looks reasonably unimportant in the context of her other responses. In any case, examining patterns of responses in the ways suggested here would be the first step in error analysis. The second step is to examine the nature of incorrect responses.

Examining the Nature of Incorrect Responses

To understand further the problem a child has, it is necessary to observe the kind of errors he or she makes. Consider another example from the Gallistel-Ellis Test of Coding Skills presented in Table 2.3. In this case, the child scores 80% on one-syllable short-vowel words with single consonants. She scores 50% on the following section, one-syllable short-vowel sounds with consonant combinations. It is

TABLE 2.3. Responses on Gallistel–Ellis Reading Test. GE Test of Coding Skills Reading–Recording Form.

	Student A					Student B				
	a	i	o	u	e	a	i	o	u	e
I. One-syllable short-vowel words with single consonants	can✓	big✓	fox✓	sun✓	red✓	can✓	big "bag"	fox✓	sun✓	red✓
	fat✓	six✓	hop✓	cup✓	yet✓	fat✓	six✓	hop "hope"	cup✓	yet✓
	pal✓	kid✓	job "jod"	hub "hud"	web "wed"	pal✓	kid✓	job✓	hub✓	web "weeb"
	jam✓	vim✓	rot✓	yum✓	peg✓	jam✓	vim✓	rot✓	yum✓	peg✓
	han✓	ziv✓	wot✓	sud✓	ket✓ 88%	han✓	ziv✓	wot "wote"	sud✓	ket✓ 80%
			Total correct 22 (25)					Total correct 20 (25)		
II. One-syllable short-vowel words with consonant combinations	that✓	kiss✓	stop✓	shut✓	help✓	that✓	kiss "kise"	stop✓	shut "shout"	help "heap"
	track✓	mint✓	strong✓	flunk✓	chest✓	track "truck"	mint✓	strong "strange"	flunk "flounk"	chest✓
	splat✓	frisk✓	prod✓	spun "spon"	smell "mell"	splat "splate"	frisk "frask"	prod "proud"	spun✓	smell✓
	cran✓	glim✓	clob✓	grum✓	ject "jest" 85%	cran✓	glim✓	clob✓	grum✓	ject 50%
			Total correct 17 (20)					Total correct 10 (20)		

tempting to conclude that she is less sure of consonant combinations and needs to be taught the process of blending, or at least specific combinations she has failed to learn. A closer look at the errors, however, indicates that the child never makes a mistake in the consonant part of the word. All of the mistakes are in the vowel. It is true that there is an apparent contradiction in this set of responses. Sometimes the child seems to know vowel sounds (Section I), and sometimes she does not (Section II). The diagnostician needs to search for an explanation through a more careful analysis of the pattern of responses, but this does not change the fact that this child knows consonant combinations.

In another example (Table 2.4), Andy has made some errors in his solution of a long division problem. His first answer is incorrect. He recognizes it and changes it to an answer that is even less appropriate. At first, his approach seems to have missed the whole point. He has no direct, efficient technique for performing the operation. However, a closer look at the nature of these errors and his approach to solution gives the diagnostician a slightly different impression. Andy has figured out a way to do long division that makes sense. He understands that multiplication is the inverse process. He even recognizes that he needs to keep track of his multiples.

Andy's problems might come under the category of what might be called "good mistakes." That is, the child begins with a basically sound principle, but either overapplies it or applies it unsystematically.

Once the nature of the errors has been identified, good or otherwise, the challenge for the diagnostician is to plan instruction. This lengthy and perhaps tedious process of error analysis has been endured because it is critical in the planning of instruction for a child with a handicap to learning. The goal has been to determine the cognitive framework from which this child operates so that it can be used to advantage as a basis for instruction. Chapter 1 emphasizes that a child's approach to the task cannot be discounted. It is the child's way of viewing the problem, and has been compiled through a series of experiences. The child has come to this approach, presumably, through a series of encounters, some of which have contributed to a valid rule system, some of which have not. The teacher or program planner must have some regard for this context. Consider,

TABLE 2.4. Andy's solution to a long division problem.

		Steps in Solution
9	(a)	452
7		$\times$ 3
$452\sqrt{34775}$	(b)	1356
		+ 452
		2808
	(d)	Counted the number of 452s to be 7
	(e)	Realized 7 is incorrect
	(f)	Recounted to 9

for example, the preschool child who is trying to remember letter sounds. The child gives correct sounds for T, B, P, D, and then explains that Y sounds like /w/. These responses imply that the child has decided on a rule for letter sounds: a letter makes the sound which is the first sound in its name. This is useful information for the teacher, since there are additional letters for which the rule does work. One approach in these circumstances would be to help the child make the rule explicit. Have the child state it or state it for him or her: "Yes, some letter sounds make . . . ." From here, instruction proceeds to include all letters and their sounds that fit this rule. Then the teacher explains that this is the extent of the rule. To drive the point home, these letters can be made into blue flash cards while nonconforming letters are otherwise color coded. At this point, a new and conflicting rule can be introduced. High contrast has the advantage of discouraging interference and erosion of the original rule. A high contrast rule might be, "Some letter sounds make the sound of the last sound in their name" – the letters F, L, M, N, R, and S can be included here. These can be assigned to red flash cards and drilled. Review of both rules and member-letter sounds can follow and, finally, the teaching of the remaining, uncategorizable letter sounds.

This method is selected to maximize the rule system that is natural to the child. The alternative is to ignore it. Under this condition, two outcomes are most likely: (1) The rule problem is not likely to go away. The child developed it for a reason. It is a *personal* formulation and has made sense to the child. It will persist and will be inappropriately applied to letter sounds such as Y. Although the rule has helped until now, with new instruction it is bound to cause an initial hindrance. (2) Another likely outcome is, after a number of instances in which the rule has not worked, the child will begin to question the original rule. This is a delicate matter. The rule is a good one. Its only deficiency is that it does not apply to all cases. This is what the child needs to understand, and this is what the suggested teaching strategy attempts to accomplish. Without such a respect for the rule, however, it is most probable that the child will reject it entirely as an inappropriate strategy. At best, the child's advantage in letter-sound learning will be lost. At worst, confusion about previously learned letter sounds as well as the ability to formulate rules will result.

In diagnostic situations, then, much, perhaps the most, is to be learned by a child's mistakes. When children err, they manage to project what is on their mind – how they are thinking about the world. In the teaching of a handicapped child, it is crucial to determine how this rule system has evolved, how it works, how it can be used to instructional advantage, how it should be avoided, and when it should be challenged.

Summary

Meaningful learning and cognitive growth cannot take place without some error production. Efforts to protect children with handicaps to learning from all error experiences seem not to be effective in enhancing any long-range goal or development. Instead, children's errors can provide a window into the idiosyncratic way their thinking and previous learning has been organized. Once a diagnostician or teacher has developed some hypothesis about the child's organizational system, it is possible to begin formulating a truly individualized approach to instruction.

3
Self-Selected Strategies

Strategic Behavior

It could be argued that all behavior is strategic. However, use of the term in the learning and memory literature has generally been limited to a type of behavior that implies specific attributes. These specifics are not always agreed upon; there is controversy regarding the extent to which the strategy must be deliberately instigated (Brown, 1975), goal directed (Paris, Newman, & Jacobs, 1985), and potentially conscious (Flavell, 1977). Pressley, Forrest-Pressley, Elliott-Faust, and Miller (1985) have discussed these elements in some detail and argue that, since strategy use can be (and arguably should be) automatized and strategies may not be consciously selected, strategic behavior need not be deliberately instigated. The following description includes all the elements that specify a useful, working definition:

A strategy is composed of cognitive operations over and above the processes that are a natural consequence of carrying out the task, ranging from one such operation to a sequence of interdependent operations. Strategies achieve cognitive purposes (e.g. comprehending, memorizing) and are potentially conscious and controllable activities (Pressley, 1982, p. 4).

For the purpose of this discussion, strategic behavior assumes the broadest definition. It includes at one extreme precise computational algorithms. At the other extreme, it allows for vaguer, heuristic processing. It includes strategies used specifically for individual content areas, such as the long division algorithm, as well as more generic, deeper levels of strategic functioning, such as attention focusing. By setting the limits of strategic behavior as broadly as possible, the likelihood of including spontaneous approaches to processing on the part of cognitively impaired children, both learning disabled and mentally retarded, is maximized.

Strategic Behavior in Cognitively Impaired
Versus Nonimpaired Populations

Strategic approaches to learning are critical for most school situations or for any other task involving symbolic material or otherwise arbitrarily associated information. In these instances, where content does not provide inherent structure, strategic behavior serves the purpose of organizing and controlling information that may have no obvious organizing features of its own. Effective learners have been found to generate a variety of strategic approaches dependent upon the nature of the task (Battig, 1975). They have some meta-awareness of the need for invoking, monitoring, evaluating, and, if necessary, modifying strategies (Brown, Bransford, Ferrara, & Campione, 1983).

There has been a fairly lengthy history of comparing strategic behavior in competent learners and in those with impairments to learning. The literature characterizes successful learners as flexible (Battig, 1975) and efficient in the production of appropriate strategies for remembering and problem solving. Children with impairments in learning, on the other hand, generally fail to generate appropriate memory and learning strategies (Belmont & Butterfield, 1971; Bray, 1979; Brown et al., 1983; Torgesen, 1980). Effective learners tend to rehearse lists (Belmont & Butterfield, 1971; Belmont, Ferretti, & Mitchell, 1982), use elaborative strategies (Campione & Brown, 1974), classify, group, or cluster information (Glidden, 1979) and, in general, devise mnemonic devices to store and access information. Noneffective learners have been characterized as passive in the face of memory tasks. They are reported not to generate appropriate mnemonic strategies spontaneously.

The body of literature that has contributed to the contrast in strategic behavior between handicapped and nonhandicapped populations consists largely of a series of studies that observe initial differences in the performance of mentally retarded or learning-disabled individuals and that of effective learners. Most methodologies proceed to an attempt to train the handicapped learners to use those strategies proven to be effective in nonhandicapped populations. Classic studies that illustrate this approach include Belmont and Butterfield's (1971) investigation of rehearsal and hesitation time patterns; Jensen and Rohwer's (1963) use of verbal mediation strategies in paired associate tasks; and Turnure and Thurlow's (1973) use of elaboration approaches. What is common in these methodologies is an effort to train mildly handicapped (in these cases educably mentally retarded) persons to use strategies that would allow for effective memory within the constraints of the particular task. A consistent finding among these studies is that performance of handicapped populations improved in the presence of experimenter-trained strategies. In fact, strategy training tends to result in equivalent performance for handicapped and nonhandicapped groups who have been equated for mental age. Nevertheless, the handicapped subjects in these studies fail to generate the same or similar strategies in the absence of direct examiner prompts.

Determinants of Strategic Behavior

The details of this literature and its methodologies are given in Chapter 4. Here the aim is to shift the focus from "exemplary" strategy usage in typical populations to spontaneous behavior in atypical populations. Much discussion has been devoted to the best fit between task and strategy choice. Less has centered around the learner × task × strategy choice interaction, Brown (1982) and Jenkins (1979) notwithstanding. This latter consideration would appear to have particular value in the study of strategic behavior in learning-disabled children, who are defined by their idiosyncratic approaches to learning.

Learning-disabled children, and to a lesser degree, mentally retarded children have specific profiles of strengths and weaknesses. They are described variously as rigid; deficient in attention processes; limited in processing capacity, short-term memory, and executive function; and a host of other descriptors. If deficient in any one of these or related areas, a child will not have the necessary resources to emulate exemplary strategies. The child's own attempts are likely to draw upon processes he or she can command or to generate imperfect copies of the model. It is possible, then, that strategies that are effective for nonhandicapped learners in their typical settings are not necessarily well suited for children with handicaps to learning or the situations in which they find themselves (Ceci & Bronfenbrenner, 1985). Since handicapped learners are defined by their inability to adapt to task demands, their profile of learning abilities and disabilities is likely to dominate despite the characteristics of the task.

Nor are task demands determined independently of learner characteristics. For example, the demands of remembering the display 8 6 5 8 9 2 3 7 are likely to be different for the person who can read large numbers and has an appreciation for place value. Such a person would be able to read these digits as one number and, thus, would place less of a burden on working memory than one who must read and remember a list of eight digits. Likewise, despite the fact that verbal mediation has been found to be an effective strategy for learning and remembering that two things are associated, a learning-disabled child who cannot access labels efficiently may not find it the most facilitative in paired-associate learning. The question of atypical learner–task interaction is an important one to raise in the effort to design or uncover effective and lasting strategies for learning in handicapped populations.

A recent study that supports the critical role of task characteristics was reported by Turner and Bray (1985). They suggest that typical memory studies, which train rehearsal strategies, involve a task that is inappropriate for handicapped individuals as well as young children. The task allows for only one exposure to the list of items to be remembered. When individuals with retardation were allowed more choice in the order and number of exposures to the list, the authors found evidence of spontaneously generated rehearsing. Such findings raise very real questions concerning the existence of spontaneous strategy usage and which strategic behaviors are likely to be generated under which conditions.

Metacognitive Passivity

The fact that preferred strategies for remembering can be elicited through training but tend not to be invoked spontaneously by mentally retarded and learning-disabled children and adults has led to the thesis that handicapped learners have a "production deficiency" (Flavell, 1977) or a metacognitive disorder (Brown, 1978; Cherkes-Julkowski, 1985). This view implies that the capacity for utilizing strategies to advantage is present and directly implicates procedures for activating strategies as the source of disorder. In pursuit of this thesis, Wong (1980) studied the incidence of inference making in learning-disabled children. Inference making and retention have been found to correlate. Wong accepts the basis of this correlation to be the role of active processing in both processes. She was able to establish that her sample of learning-disabled children from grades 2 to 6 did not spontaneously construct inferences. Nevertheless, when probed with additional questioning, in the absence of any further instruction or exposure to the information, learning-disabled children did evidence inferential reasoning. In our clinical work with learning-disabled children, we have found a similar tendency. When asked to summarize a story just read or heard, learning-disabled children generally offer cursory descriptions. When asked, "Anything else?" repeatedly, the story usually unfolds in considerable depth and detail. There seems, then, to be a generalized lack of active organizing and retrieving behavior.

Further support for a subgroup of learning-disabled children who might be classified as passive comes from a series of studies reported by Torgesen, by Tarver, and by Hallahan. These children have been shown to benefit from strategy training (Dawson, Hallahan, Reeve, & Ball, 1980), but failed to apply those strategies in similar but novel situations. Although incentives tended to improve memory performance in learning-disabled children (Haines & Torgesen, 1979; Hallahan, Tarver, Kauffman, & Graybeal, 1979), there was no evidence that incentives increased the use of mnemonic strategies (Gelabert, Torgesen, Dice, & Murphy, 1980). There is some evidence, then, that atypical learners have an available store of strategies, but cannot or do not activate them when they are needed. To pursue the computer analogy often applied to metacognition, this population does not execute the appropriate program for processing information, or it is lacking in the executive function itself.

Misguided Attention

Although the passivity of handicapped populations in the face of specific learning and memory tasks has been generally accepted, the source of that passivity remains the subject of some discussion. It has been argued that the essence of the difficulty lies in selective and active attention. Accordingly, handicapped learners are described as unable to weed out extraneous, incidental, or irrelevant information in order to focus actively on those dimensions of the task that are critical to its comprehension (Zeaman & House, 1963a, 1963b, 1979). Instead of selecting critical features for attention, handicapped learners are likely at one extreme to accept incidental features as significant aspects of an event or object (Hupp, Conroy, & Able, 1986). At the other extreme, responses of ineffective learners have been characterized as task welded (Brown et al., 1983; Burger, Blackman, Clark, & Gordon, 1982; Cherkes-Julkowski, 1985); that is, all features are accepted as relevant rather than only the critical ones, and all must be reexperienced to trigger an association. The latter approach prohibits the selection of critical features that form the foundation for categorization generalization (Rosch, 1977).

Differences in selective attention occur as early as the fifth month of life (Caron & Caron, 1981; Witelson, 1977). In contrast to full-term infants, preterm infants who are at risk for learning disabilities or developmental delay tend to disregard invariant features of a relationship or the defining configuration that overrides the mere elements of a visual display. Instead, they attend to the discrete components of the content. Although they differ in what they find salient or critical in the display, preterm and full-term infants are similar in the amount of attention given and the ability to make discriminations based on that to which they have attended.

There has been some experimentation with encouraging handicapped learners to attend more carefully to the critical aspects of the task. In these studies, no further problem-solving or metacognitive aids are provided. Both Feuerstein (1980) and Budoff and Corman (1976) report significant gains after such treatment. According to Feuerstein and his associates (Burns et al., 1983), the act of helping a learner focus attention to the task constitutes a mediated learning experience, a learning experience that is guided by another, a parent or teacher, and that directs the child to the critical features in the environment. Children who have been given the opportunity to have mediated learning experiences are more likely to have developed a set for learning through attention tuning and through indirect learning in the form of reception of information about the environment from others. Typically, the role of mediator is assumed during infancy and preschool by the parent or caregiver and is relinquished gradually as the child assumes responsibility for the regulation of his or her own task-orienting processes (Hodapp, Goldfield, & Boyatzis, 1984; Wertsch, Minick, & Arns, 1984). Learning-disabled students have been found to be particularly amenable to interventions that assist them in attention focusing (Haywood, 1977).

Knowledge Structure and Attention

Caron and Caron (1981) suggest a different approach to modifying attention in vulnerable infants. They emphasize the importance of experience with multiple exemplars. Only by such variations on a theme does the theme assume a central role. The ability to determine which aspects of a task or problem are critical and thus warrant the focus of attention, then, depends at least in part on how much one already knows about the world, its regularity, its customs, and its conventions. In developmentally young children, one would expect a lesser accumulation of knowledge. Mervis (1984) points out that in addition to greater naivete, young children notice, store information, and construct their knowledge networks based on what is salient to them. She distinguishes between adult-basic and child-basic categories. The latter are based on perceptual similarities and are relatively unaffected by issues of function or convention. For example, Mervis describes the tendency of toddlers to include a spherical candle, a spherical piggy bank, and a ball into the single category of ball. It is not until the child notices or is assisted in noticing the candle wick or the bank slot for coins that the different function of these items, and therefore their membership in another class based on function, can be explained.

Just as the young child has an idiosyncratic approach to classifying objects and events, so does a child with a history of cognitive impairments. Such children have built their knowledge structure on a series of experiences influenced by what they have found salient, based on their processing mechanisms. Knowledge structure, then, is not independent of strategic or processing behavior. They define each other. What one addresses as salient determines the classification scheme of the knowledge store and thus what one is likely to recognize as salient in the future. Little work has been done in the effort to examine the nature of knowledge structures in impaired versus competent learners. More attention, however, has been given to knowledge structures in naive versus expert subjects (Chi, 1978) and some to knowledge structures in high versus low achievers in a given content area (Donald, 1982). These efforts establish the real difference in the way knowledge is stored in those who are more versus those less experienced or accomplished in a given area. The differences promise to be more extreme when impaired and competent learners are contrasted.

The more a child has been able to learn about his or her world and the more elaborate the connections among stored information points, the more likely the child is to recognize critical features and approximations of prototypes (Rosch, 1977). What a learner already knows is not, then, independent of what he or she is able to notice about a novel situation. Likewise, prior knowledge is not independent of how one processes information in a novel setting. Chi and Koeske (1983) have established that the amount of information stored in one's knowledge structure as well as the quality of the network of associations among information points or nodes determines, at least in part, how much is to be learned and in what way. An experienced chess player (Chi, 1978), for example, will be able to include more information about the board in a single encounter than will a novice player. Since the capacity for processing information is finite (Miller, 1956), the degree to which the richness and integrity of the knowledge structure maximizes or diminishes capacity is critical. Along this dimension, handicapped learners are likely to be disadvantaged in several ways. Many have been placed in learning environments that narrow their exposure to a smaller number of controlled experiences. Regardless of exposure, learning rate is almost certainly slower than that of nonhandicapped groups. In addition, handicapped learners have been characterized as having a structurally more limited capacity (Case, 1978; Spitz, 1966). Each of these constraints, either separately or in combination, alters typical attention focusing processes.

Context and Attention

Gibson and Rader (1979) speak of vigilance in attending. They explain that young children and some handicapped older children are unable to maintain an active focus to achieve a specific goal. For most preschool children or for children in nonliterate societies (Charlesworth, 1976; Olsen, 1976), the need for active and vigilant attention is diminished; that is, symbol-free situations that occur in context carry an integrated message. The situation dramatizes those elements that play critical roles and tends to demonstrate the insignificance of lesser ones. Elements in the situation have natural relationships to each other. Learning of this kind and in these kinds of situations is what Piaget describes in the developing child and what has led him, as well as others (Siegler, 1978), to characterize preschoolers as young scientists. The role of child is to observe and experiment, but ultimately to receive and accept natural laws or rules within recurring physical or social situations (Gelman & Spelke, 1981). In addition to being pre-organized, systematic, and integrated, context-bound situations of these kinds are often self-selected. A young preschool child is apt to pursue something of personal choice that follows from an immediate need or curiosity. All of these factors contribute to a reduced need to focus attention actively or to find some way to impose a strategy for making sense out of a given situation.

Symbol learning, learning of information out of context, or learning of information that has been selected by someone else requires a different approach to the task. No observable laws determine that the configuration "b" is called "B" and that it has the sound associated with the initial sound in *bat*. The learning of these associations requires some activity, even vigilance, on the part of the learner, who must realize first that this is one of those situations that requires something more than observing and collecting data that are bound to fall into place. The learner will need to find some way to decide which elements of the letter are critical. For this purpose, it will be necessary to recognize that directionality is important. Thus, a "b" is not a "d." The learner will be required further to find some way to remember the name and sound of both, which are arbitrarily associated with this configuration. Together, these goals require mnemonic strategies and active selection of relevant dimensions.

Studies with very young children accentuate the effect of natural context on learning and memory behavior. When a child 9 months of age is asked to remember under which cup an object is hidden, he or she is more likely to be able to do so in familiar settings. In fact, at home the 9-month-old can observe the hiding of an object, then be rotated 180° to the other side of the table where the object and cups have been placed, and can identify even with this new left–right orientation where the object is. In an unfamiliar laboratory, this level of performance was not attained (Acredolo, 1978). In a series of reports, DeLoache (1980, 1984) also indicates the facilitative effects of familiar, natural contexts on remembering, this time in toddlers ranging in age from 18 to 23 months. In her studies, children were asked to watch where a toy was hidden, to wait, and to retrieve it at a later time. At home this task presented little difficulty. In the lab, performance was significantly diminished. DeLoache (1980) argues that memory in the context of natural environments requires little strategy production. The arrangement of the environment provides so many associations and cues that the need for self-generated associations is reduced. It is enough to recognize that the toy is under the pillow. That the pillow is on the couch, the couch next to the table, and so on, is a part of a well-learned, integrated network of associations.

Despite, or perhaps because of, the toddler's relative ease of remembering in natural environments, his or her use of strategic behaviors in unfamiliar settings is proportionately greater. In the lab setting for the hide and seek game, toddlers verbalized more about the toy and its hiding place, looked, pointed, and approached frequently (DeLoache & Brown, 1983). DeLoache (1984) goes on to report, however, that there is no significant correlation between the frequency of strategy usage and accurate toy retrieval. The lack of relationship between strategy production and effective recall might be explained by the fact that strategy production is more frequent in exactly those situations where recall is most difficult. Despite the possible (and probable) facilitating effects of mnemonic strategies, their presence indicates that memory will be difficult. In contrast, Krupski (1985) has reported that handicapped children demonstrate fewer active task attending behaviors as cognitive demands increase. It is primarily in those situations with the greatest demand for active strategy production that handicapped learners are apt to retreat.

Comparisons of this kind between strategy usage in handicapped versus non-handicapped learners are difficult to make. Nonhandicapped learners are seldom studied in relationship to handicapped learners on tasks that are exceptionally difficult for them. It is possible that a U-shaped curve describes the amount of strategic behavior in both populations; that is, at some optimal level of task difficulty, strategic behavior would be at its peak. Beyond this point, due to the overwhelming demands of the task, fewer active attempts would be made.

The relationship between behaviors and familiarity with the environment has been reported among school-age children at 10 and 14 years old as well (Ceci & Bronfenbrenner, 1985). Children in this study were asked to bake cupcakes at home in their own kitchen and in a lab-based kitchen. Their task was to place the cupcakes in the oven at a specified time and to remove them 30 min later. In the interval they were invited to play a video game. At home, children manifested an efficient and systematic strategy for time monitoring. In the lab, the children who were able to remove the cupcakes at the correct time needed to check the time more frequently, less systematically, and more "anxiously." Those in the lab who failed to adopt a strategy of overmonitoring tended to let the cupcakes go too long. Ceci and Bronfenbrenner (1985) emphasize the facilitative effects of a familiar environment in producing fairly complex strategies in an automatic way. In unfamiliar settings some cognitive space and energy is required to collect new information about the environment and to make new associations among and about information points. Novel situations require more involved strategy usage for the management of new information as well as for the function of creating cognitive capacity for the assigned task.

Vagueness, Imprecision, and Strategic Behavior

The discussion thus far has focused on the presence or absence of spontaneously generated strategies in handicapped learners. Recent investigation into memory and retrieval processes in learning-disabled children (Howe, Brainerd, & Kingma, 1985) suggests that differences between handicapped and nonhandicapped persons may be something more than just quantitative. Howe and colleagues (1985) make a distinction between algorithmic and heuristic retrieval processes: "Specifically, algorithmic retrieval is any errorless recall operation, whereas heuristic retrieval is any operation that produces item recall on some trials but fails to do so on others" (p. 1123). Results indicate that learning-disabled children tend to use heuristic operations as well as nonhandicapped children of the same chronologic age, but do not employ precise algorithmic retrieval processes as reliably.

The characterization of strategies employed by the learning disabled as imprecise and vague is supported in other lines of research as well. Learning-disabled students have been found to be less apt to use organizational strategies than the nonhandicapped (Dallago & Moely, 1980; Wong, Wong, & Foth, 1977). In our study of learning-disabled junior college students (McGuire, Cherkes-Julkowski, & Gertner, 1985), we found a similarly vague and loosely controlled set of problem-solving strategies. Learning-disabled students were asked, as one part of this study, to solve two of the Block Design tasks on the Wechsler Adult Intelligence Scales (WAIS). The achievement of a correct versus an incorrect response was of less interest than observations of spontaneously generated strategies. The Block Design task was selected over more obviously verbal tasks because the necessity to provide a motor response made it possible to observe strategies, partial solutions, and error patterns. Subjects were asked to estimate the difficulty and time requirements of each of the two designs prior to beginning the reproduction of each. After each design was completed, subjects were given feedback about the amount of time a correct replication took or were told that their design had not been completed. A primary concern in the study was (1) performance on the second block design after students had been asked to focus on the difficulty of task 1 and thus, indirectly, the demands of this kind of task; and (2) had been given feedback about their performance and the accuracy of their evaluation concerning its difficulty. In addition to the learning-disabled students, low-achieving and normally achieving junior college students were asked to perform the same task. Low-achieving students were selected to match the achievement level of the learning-disabled group. Normally achieving students were selected to match the full-scale aptitude scores of the learning-disabled group. Discriminant function analysis based on block design approaches could differentiate among the three groups with a high degree of accuracy (96.97%). None of the measures concerning performance on the design completed first, along or in combination with other measures, was able to differentiate among the three groups. Three measures of strategy usage on the second design completed, however, comprised the discriminant functions derived. Low-achieving junior college students made a greater number of total errors on their second design than both normally achieving and learning-disabled groups. The ratio of correct to incorrect moves was similar for low-achieving and learning-disabled students. Both scores reflected an error rate twice as high as that of the normally achieving group. An informative distinction between learning-disabled and low-achieving students appeared in the comparison of correct initial placements changed to incorrect placements. Learning-disabled students changed a greater number of initially correct placements than did either of the other groups. In contrast, the low-achieving students appeared to be aware of a correct placement once performed despite a relatively unplanful, trial and error approach.

Despite the lack of precision in their approach to task completion and performance monitoring, the learning-disabled students demonstrated some ability to evaluate task demands. Errors on the first task are related to estimates of difficulty on the second and to time requirements on both the first and second designs. The relationship between task evaluation and actual performance in low-achieving students is neither as consistent nor as strong. The typical low-achieving student does manifest some degree of post-task awareness of demands, but does not seem to apply it in the pretask evaluation of the next very highly related problem. Learning-disabled students are much better at this process, but continue to evince imprecise, vague strategies that fail to recognize the correctness of partial solutions. This pattern is consistent with Howe, Brainerd, and Kingmas' (1985) portrayal of the learning-disabled child who tends to use strategies for learning and remembering that do not reflect a systematic, algorithmic approach, but rather suggest a loosely connected, fuzzy system of task solution.

It should be noted that imprecise and vague or fuzzy concepts or rule systems are not unique to handicapped individuals. This kind of thinking has been found to characterize language and concept development during the early stages of all development. When a child is first beginning to say words (somewhere around 15 to 18 months of age) he or she is likely to overgeneralize or overextend their application (Brown, 1958). Thus, all four-legged animals are called "horsies." Overgeneralizations are certainly evident in young children, but are not uncommon in school-age children or even in adults. At any age an individual's initial understanding of a new concept is characterized by a vague notion that becomes refined only gradually through experience (Mervis, 1984; Rosch, 1977; Zadeh, 1982). According to this view, initial concept formation involves the development of a prototype. A prototype is derived from a series of examples from a given class of objects (Rosch, 1977; Zadeh, 1982). A prototype is neither a single best example nor a collection of good examples, but rather a more or less fuzzy scheme that represents a cross section of exemplars and can serve to generate other instances of the category. According to prototype theory it becomes possible, then, to decide whether something is an example of a particular class and the degree to which it is a good example. It is not possible, however, to provide explicit rules that define the class or determine its exemplars. It is the very fuzziness of developing concepts that allows for their extension as well as their overextension.

On the continuum from extremely fuzzy processing to extreme precision there is an optimal level of each that is likely to vary according to the nature of the task. As is the case with most developmental phenomena, a U-shaped growth curve is likely to be most descriptive (Karmiloff-Smith, 1981; Strauss, 1982; Thelen, 1986). In a well-titled article, "If You Want to Get Ahead, Get a Theory," Karmiloff-Smith and Inhelder (1974/75) suggest that the first level of processing involves formulating a broad, overinclusive approach analogous to a fuzzy set. Once the set or theory is operative, one can begin to use it and, as a result of feedback from the environment, continue to hone and refine it. During this testing period, children or adults are likely to seem to be regressing. Where they appeared to know something earlier, they now tend to apply concepts or rules erroneously. Karmiloff-Smith defends this as a critical step in testing the limits and constructing a more precise and ruleful understanding.

Concepts or rule systems, then, are refined gradually through the process of defining negative instances of those objects that do not belong to the class. This is the goal in scientific thinking (Kuhn, 1977). To test a theory, one must search for counterexamples or disproving instances of it. This is not an easy or a natural process. In a series of studies with adult college students, Wason and his colleagues (Wason & Johnson-Laird, 1972a, 1972b) have identified an "obsessive tendency" to develop a rule and to defend it at any cost. Rather than look for contradictions or even accept them when they are demonstrated, adults prefer to maintain their original conceptualization and to insist that it is correct and workable. Contradictions are treated as if they are irrelevant.

Fuzzy schemes and overextensions, therefore, are not simply associated with errors or impaired learning processes. They are natural at all stages of development. In the stages of learning model proposed by Howe and colleagues (1985), an imprecise, heuristic approach to retrieval is found typically in nonhandicapped learners during the initial stages of problem attack. The failure of handicapped learners to progress beyond this point, to derive secondary, more precise algorithms when they are needed, seems at least in part due to passivity. That is, rather than actively sort out conflicting data, it remains less unsettling to retain one's initial conceptualization or rule system, however vague. Learning-disabled children are described as easily confused and disorganized (Strauss & Lehtinen, 1947). It would be especially attractive for them to avoid confusion. Cawley (personal communication) reported an anecdote that illustrates just such a distaste for confusion. He was attempting to develop a reading comprehension test that eliminated the opportunity for correct comprehension answers based in previously learned information rather than the currently read passage. To do this, he invented nonsense sentences such as, "The baby was robbing eggs from the robin" and asked learning-disabled as well as normally achieving elementary school children to point to a picture of the just-read sentence. He found it difficult to involve the learning-disabled youngsters in the task. They were uncomfortably confused and stated strongly that they did not want to continue. In contrast, the normally achieving group enjoyed the task, which they found humorous.

Vague, heuristic, or wholistic processing of this kind has been associated with right- versus left-brain activity (Kaufman & McLean, 1986; Zaidel, 1979). The right brain is associated with approaches that derive configurational rather than detailed, sequential analyses. Failure to go beyond the level of configurational, general, fuzzy analysis may merely reflect differences in cognitive style or, more gravely, disorders related to left brain functions. It is interesting to consider, in this light, that the vast majority of learning-disabled children are identified on the basis of language and reading disorders that would reflect problems with functions processed primarily in the left brain.

A typical finding among learning-disabled children with reading problems is their tendency to read whole words as if they were configurations, rather than composed of distinct sequences of letters to be decoded systematically. These children are likely to read *price* as *prince*, *kitten* as *kitchen*, or *could* as *cloud* when words are presented out of context. There is a great deal of debate about what kinds of processing facilitate or inhibit competent decoding in reading, (Mann, 1986) including contributions made by linguistic awareness and auditory as opposed to visual memory. Regardless of the source, the error of whole-word approximation is reminiscent of fuzzy, unanalyzed rather than systematic, methodical, and explicit processing.

In a symbol system where graphemes represent phonemes depending on their position in relationship to other graphemes and where each symbol is critical to decoding, explicit and, in this case, sequential analysis is vital. This kind of explicit approach, however, is not optimal in all situations or at all steps in the learning process. There are situations in which there is simply too much information, too many organizing themes to capture in a limited-capacity system. In such situations the competent, flexible learner would be able to relinquish strategies for precise analysis, relying instead on processing receptive to patterns, themes, or correlated features in the stimulus situation.

There are dangers and benefits to each approach, and each can enhance the other if counterbalanced appropriately. The appeal of explicit, rule-based processing is its capacity for reducing information processing to reliable, universal principles that can be worked and applied in a multitude of situations. The advantage in terms of clarity as well as economy is clear from the perspective of spontaneous processing or of instructing children in rules to be used as a basis for processing. At the same time, economy can be achieved at the expense of complexity. Economy is achieved by deriving a frame or rule for focusing on critical, defining features and thus alleviating the need to scan for additional information. Shweder (1977) stresses that it is the need for manageability and comfort in cognitive operations that leads people to deal in stereotypes about groups of others rather than in terms of idiosyncracies and variance in behavior.

The reality is, however, that few rules have universal application. The sound of "a" in *cat* is not the same as in pat or cap. The final vowel "e" signals a different rule in *hose* than in *house* (Weir & Venezky, 1968). Where is the rule that explains *lemon* versus *demon* and *know*, *no*, *now*, and *known*? There is a group of learning-disabled children and young adults (McGuire et al., 1985) who seem to be overrulified. They tend to overmonitor their strategies in an effort to consider all the possible rules that might apply and to decide on the most appropriate. The result is often overload, overstimulation, and ultimately retreat. This tendency to monitor to a fault could be part of an inadequate metacognitive system in the first place. However, it might owe at least some of its existence to instruction designed to make rules explicit, learnable, and generalizable, as well as to lack of confidence. Again, the suggestion is not that no instruction about explicit rules should take place. It is only that some balance must be found between controlled versus more implicit processing.

Some concepts or relationships simply cannot be driven to a series of explicit formulas. At advanced stages of reading skill acquisition, this is true (e.g., lemon/demon). It is true at the level of basic concept formation. Certainly very young children can group different kinds of apples together and differentiate them from pears as well as from other fruit (Rosch, 1977). Neither they nor adults are able to provide explicit defining principles for what is intended by appleness or for what distinguishes that concept from pearness. In the case of concept formation in young children or in the early stages of acquisition at any age, very first awareness seems to be at an implicit, unanalyzed level. Such an awareness might be recognized as a template, prototype, set, or frame (Brooks, 1978) for organizing information about the world. The frame, then, enables a more efficient means for scanning the environment for additional information relevant for its growth and modification (Karmiloff-Smith, 1981). As more information is collected and the boundaries of the frame/concept become better delineated, clarity about what is included and excluded begins to be achieved. Of particular value in this process are encounters with negative examples or contradictions (Piaget, 1970; Wason & Johnson-Laird, 1972a, 1972b; Zimmerman & Blom, 1983), which serve the purpose of making explicit those properties of the frame that are not valid and, conversely, those that are. Explicit or perhaps literal awareness is operative until, as discussed earlier, the information load becomes too great. Then, a more resilient, less stress-prone system of implicit processing would be required again. And, thus, it would proceed ad infinitum.

In our clinical observations with learning-disabled youngsters, we have found that it is quite difficult to make this shift. Some children with low scores on either performance (Wechsler, 1974) or simultaneous (Kaufman & Kaufman, 1983) functions may lack the capacity generally associated with areas in the right hemisphere of the brain for working at an implicit level. Similarly, low verbal (Wechsler, 1974) or sequential (Kaufman & Kaufman, 1983) scores might suggest difficulties with explicit, regulating functions of the left hemisphere. There are children, however, who are weak in neither subscale of the WISC-R or the Kaufman Assessment Battery for Children (Kaufman & Kaufman, 1983) but who still demonstrate a wide discrepancy between the two scales, perhaps 25 to 30 points. These are very bright youngsters who tend to score perhaps 110 on one scale and 135 on the other. Our experience has been with children whose strengths are in performance/simultaneous areas, most probably because they are screened out due to the verbal, sequential demands of school instruction. These children would not appear on the surface to have any kind of disability. Our observations, however, indicate a strong trend on the part of these children to be unable to make the shift from implicit to explicit analysis. This is perhaps best illustrated in a quote from a 13-year-old boy with the following profile:

Detroit Tests of Learning Aptitude–2 (1985)*

Conceptual Matching	16
Word Opposites	14
Sentence Imitation	9
Word Sequences	7
Object Sequences	5

*Standard scores have a mean of 10 and a standard deviation of 3.

Wechsler Intelligence Scale for Children–Revised (1974)[†]

Information	16	Picture Completion	19
Arithmetic	16	Block Design	13
Digit Span	4	Coding	9

[†] Scaled scores have a mean of 10 and a standard deviation of 3.

Raven Test of Progressive Matrices (1949)

95th percentile

When asked to provide a writing sample, he produced the following passage:

My science teacher gets a new program. He can't figure it out. He goes to sleep, next mornin' he wakes up and he does it. Yesterday Dr. _____ (school psychologist) gave me a puzzle to do (WISC-R, Block Design). I couldn't figure it out. This mornin' I woke up figured it out.

Included here as well is an excerpt from the educational evaluation:

The best description of this child's cognitive style can be found in his own account of solving the WISC-R Block Design. He does not impose frames for organizing information on stimuli he confronts. Instead he seems to remain in a completely receptive state. As a result he absorbs a great deal of information but fails to systematize it in order to avoid overload and in order to have a more controlled command over what he has encountered. One manifestation of this is the inability to provide a clear verbal description for his correct Raven solutions. The very real advantage to this child's style is a tremendous fluidity and depth of understanding as well as a potential for creativity. The disadvantage is that he lacks any resistance to the inflow of information. This child's cognitive style prepares him particularly well for creating fuzzy sets which have great potential for concept acquisition, transfer and analogical thinking. His style is particularly ill-equipped for capturing a rapid flow of relatively disconnected information. This child seems unprepared to formulate frames for organizing or systematizing information for the sheer purpose of compressing information so that it can be managed more efficiently. Instead he maintains an effort to absorb everything until a deeper meaning becomes apparent and itself provides a more essential organizing frame. Ironically, it is exactly this form of processing in which this child is weak which is most critical during the initial stages of learning or coping with any new situation. This places this child in a situation in which, unless he is very resilient, he is out before he is in.

Although this child's achievement scores are within grade level, his inability to meet with school demands is real as is evidenced in his nearly failing grades and poor school adjustment. His inability is at least in part based in cognitive deficiencies characterized by lack of controlled strategies for managing information. Since working memory is where these strategies are most essential, it is in this area that the child manifests extreme weakness. The discrepancy between his very poor performance in working memory and his superior performance in abstract reasoning (Raven) as well as concept formation (conceptual matching on the Detroit−2) spans more than 3 standard deviations. This child seems clearly in need of support services in order to develop strategies for dealing with extreme cognitive strengths and weaknesses as well as for adapting to the kind of learning required in school.

Environmental Contribution to Passivity and Imprecision

Regardless of one's motivation for or capacity to work through confusion to a more precise rule system, confusion or conflict resolution is a necessary condition for achieving a higher cognitive level (Piaget, 1970). Unless a rule is formulated and extended a learner will neither be able to manage the large amounts of information in any one display or be able to test hypotheses. For example, at first a young child might assume that all past tense verbs are marked by an *ed* ending. The child proceeds to construct words accordingly. Environmental feedback for normally developing children tends to allow lawful errors of this kind for awhile (Mervis, 1984). Then, it begins to provide information about adult-level standards for performance. In this way the U-shaped curve is acted out. The environment responds differently to vulnerable children, especially those who appear passive or noninitiating from birth. There is a large literature concerning the intrusive, highly directive quality of mothers' behaviors toward Down's syndrome (Jones, 1980; Mervis, 1984) and preterm (Rocissano & Yatchmink, 1983) infants and toddlers. Maternal directiveness seems due at least partially to a desire to protect developing children from errors that will impede steady growth along a linear hierarchy. Mothers and teachers of infants who are handicapped or at risk seem determined to avoid the dip in the U-shaped curve. According to almost any theory of cognitive development, however, this is an ill-conceived approach to fostering growth. Without self-generated errors, rule systems remain unclarified and imprecise.

Stern and Hildebrandt (1986) suggest that parents create the passive, stereotyped behavior associated with the learning-disabled and mildly retarded school-age child. In their effort to overprotect their young children from error-prone behavior, they impose adult-level systems (Mervis, 1984) from the beginning, thereby discouraging the child from generating his or her own self-generated rules for categorizing information about the world. This approach is perpetuated by school programs that vow to provide "successful," error-free approaches to learning. The vulnerable child, then, seems born into a system of transactions between self and environment that encourage passivity. Handicapped learners seem unable to go beyond this to the ability to formulate and reformulate continually more precise strategies even at later stages in the learning process.

Spontaneous Strategy Generation

In an effort to describe how handicapped learners formulate strategies when encouraged to do so or when they were at least not impeded in their effort, we have conducted a series of studies. In the preliminary study of strategy usage in cognitively impaired children that served as the pilot for the study reported in detail in Chapter 5, we asked children to work in teams of three to discuss the best way to remember things. Groups of learning-disabled children were distinct in their approach to this task. They tended to use what the study termed *overextended elaborations*, characterized by story telling that went far afield from the original stimulus items. For example, when asked to remember that a picture of an apple was to be associated with a picture of a girl, three learning-disabled children aged 7 years, IQ 100, held the following discussion:

C: The girl's after the apple, trips on the apple because it's in the way.
T: There is a worm in the apple (the picture has a mark that could be interpreted as a hole).
C: When the husky comes and eats the apple, the worm's going to blast his head.
T: The apple falls on her head and knocks her out.
C: The helicopter bombs the husky and knocks her out.
T: A helicopter comes by and shoots a bow and arrow into it.
C: Firing missiles, sledge hammer knocks her out.
D: Apple's throwing seeds at it.
T: She spits the seeds out of the apple.
C: She goes by the pool and the apple comes and pushes her in backwards and she drowns.

Data analysis indicated that despite the appearance of excessive imprecision and distractibility, the use of overextended elaborations (our somewhat mislabeled term) of this type was strongly associated with good memory performance for learning-disabled children and for slow learners, but not for averagely functioning children. Although it is not an original finding that elaborations (Pressley, 1982; Turnure & Thurlow, 1973) can facilitate memory and deep processing (Bransford, 1979; Johnson-Laird, 1983), previous research indicates the failure of cognitively impaired children to construct elaborations or to deep process on their own. One critical difference in the design of this study in contrast to most others is the lack of experimenter-imposed elaborations, as well as the design of a peer group intended to facilitate self- and peer-generated strategies. The design of the actual study and final results are reported in Chapter 6.

In contrast to the kind of elaborations used by learning-disabled children consider this discussion, by three gifted second graders, of the best way to remember the pairing of a cross shape and a quarter-moon shape:

P: That looks like a satellite (cross) and that looks like a moon.
 I: That does not look like a satellite, it looks like a red cross, that could be a hospital or an ambulance.
C: Yeah.
P: But if you call that a cross you won't remember it goes with the moon.
 I: Maybe it's a star. It could look kind of like a star.
P: Now at least you're out in space.

These children remain focused on the need to create a clear connection between the pictures. As a group, they refine their labeling to remain within the limits of the connecting relationship, "out in space." The ability to steer the discussion efficiently toward the central theme in this group is quite different from the athematic wanderings of the learning-disabled group. There is a long tradition in the field of special education and other kinds of remedial programs of identifying "good" strategies for learning, those used by competent children. Nevertheless, evidence is beginning to collect suggesting that this is not a workable approach. First, the approach bears little if any fruit at the stage of generalization (Brown et al., 1983). Furthermore, handicapped learners come to a task with their own set of abilities and disabilities that redefine what is good and workable and what is not (Wachs, 1985). For example, in the preliminary study of strategy usage cited earlier (Cherkes-Julkowski et al., 1986), it was found that a qualitatively different pattern of strategy usage was associated with memory performance for each of the three groups studied—slow learners, learning-disabled, and normally achieving children. The exact nature of these findings will be discussed more thoroughly in Chapter 6. Further support for differential paths to competent performance can be found in our ongoing longitudinal study of preterm and full-term development (Cherkes-Julkowski, Foley, Davis, Marrion, & Roth, 1985). Preliminary analyses reveal that qualitatively different sets of variables at 2, 5, and 8 months predict outcomes at 10 months in the two groups studied.

"Good" Strategies Redefined

An approach to intervention that attempts to impose "good strategies" on handicapped learners, then, does not seem a likely approach to effective instruction. There are, apparently, no "good strategies." There are only those strategies that facilitate learning for particular individuals or groups of individuals. Since learning-disabled youngsters are expected to have specific patterns of strengths and weaknesses in learning, they would be particularly sensitive to strategies that impose an approach to problem solving that interferes with a preferred or compensatory one.

In the first of our investigations into the processes of strategy usage and strategy selections in handicapped learners, we studied the possibility that suggesting that a learner must choose among a set of strategies would transfer to strategy usage in an unprompted situation and would increase memory performance

(Cherkes-Julkowski et al., 1986). The rationale for this approach is founded in a review of previous methodologies. By far, the predominant method for studying strategy usage in handicapped populations is either through setting task restraints and comparing nonhandicapped and handicapped persons equated for mental or chronological age (Belmont & Butterfield, 1971; Turner & Bray, 1985) or both, or through training the handicapped population in a single "good" strategy for remembering. For example, studies of paired-associate learning have trained handicapped persons to use verbal mediation strategies (Jensen & Rohwer, 1963; Turnune & Thurlow, 1973) or elaboration strategies (Campione & Brown, 1974). To enhance serial learning, investigators have trained the handicapped to use rehearsal strategies (Butterfield, Wambold, & Belmont, 1973). Advance organizers have been used to facilitate memory of a connected narrative (Peleg & Moore, 1982). In all of these lines of research, however, one strategy is trained. Most studies proceed to test for maintenance of strategy usage over time. Two weeks is a typical delay period. Finally, the ability to generate the trained strategy on a novel set of stimuli is tested. Even maintenance is hard to establish in these studies, although extensive overtraining and brief relearning episodes have been found to be effective (Kellas, Ashcraft, & Johnson, 1973). Generalization has been virtually impossible to elicit (Brown et al., 1983; Butterfield et al., 1973; Jensen & Rohwer, 1963). Several explanations have been offered for these repeated findings, varying from a nonremedial deficit in generalization per se to problems of task analysis resulting in inadequate evaluation of the near/far quality required by experimenter-derived tasks (Belmont & Butterfield, 1977).

We considered the possibility that every stimulus situation was, at least in some way, slightly different from every other. All changes in stimuli would require some modification in the strategy or strategies used to respond to them. Under these conditions, training on single-strategy usage would be likely to introduce some hazards. It is possible that such an experimental intervention would serve the purpose of creating the expectation that a single, unmodifiable strategy was a viable procedure for the solution of all memory-related tasks.

At the very least, then, single-strategy training might provide a counterproductive set for failing to adapt to stimulus demands. This thesis suggests particular difficulty in generalization tasks where the stimuli are different and experimenter prompts are not provided. This, of course, is exactly what research has shown to be true. Additional problems in single-strategy training might be implicated among the learning disabled. If it is true that learning-disabled persons prefer distinct strategies over others and that one learning-disabled person's performance might be facilitated by strategies quite different from the next, the hazards of training a "best" strategy become that much more apparent.

We pursued the idea that it seemed counterproductive to encourage the notion in handicapped learners that one strategy could suffice for most problems. Instead, what appeared to be critical was an improved capacity to select from among a variety of task-related strategies. Our study required learning-disabled, slow-learning, and normally achieving school-age children from the ages of 6 to 15 years to remember pairs of pictures.

Three sets of paired-stimulus pictures were designed. Each pair consisted of line drawings on 3 × 5 laminated cards. Each set of eight paired stimuli was intended to appeal to a different strategy for memorizing and recalling the second member of a pair. The three strategies included the following:

1. *Similarity–semantic paring strategy.* Each pair of pictured common objects in this set could be combined under a common classification (i.e., a tulip and a daisy would be paired under a single semantic label of flowers; similarly, a bird in flight and a perched bird would be paired under the semantic label of birds). Thus, the task required something more than simple matching. It appealed to the use of a single label to aid memory of both items.
2. *Sentential verbal mediation strategy.* Totally unrelated pairs of common objects were selected so that they could be linked in a simple sentence, "The _____ is on the _____." Typically, these objects would not be found "on" each other. The use of the sentence mediator was intended to facilitate memory and recall.
3. *Rehearsal strategy.* Pairs of abstract nonrepresentational forms were developed as stimuli that did not readily lend themselves to simple classification (semantic pairing) or simple labeling for linkage in a sentence (sentential mediations). Nonrepresentational forms were used to discourage semantic or sentential associations between the items in a pair. Training procedures modeled the process of generating a label for those forms and rehearsing that label.

See Figures A.1 and A.3 in the Appendix.

Each child was pretested to establish that he or she could perform a memory task and command the task of pointing to the correct picture, which would be required in the experimental situation. Next, children were assigned to treatment groups. Each group of children was trained on two of the three strategies used in the study.

Each subject, then, received either semantic/sentential, semantic/rehearsal, or rehearsal/sentential training. Within each training subgroup, half of the subjects were trained in one order (e.g., sentential first, rehearsal second). The other half were trained in the reverse order.

In each training condition, each subject was told the experimenter was going to give him or her a trick to aid memory. Each subject was then given a sample trial. For the similarities condition, instructions consisted of the experimenter placing two pictures in a vertical row facing the subject and explaining: "Here's the trick. These (experimenter points to each picture) are the same things. Same things go together. Now remember." Following this explanation the experimenter removed the pictures, replaced the stimulus picture, and presented a card with an array of nine pictures including the appropriate response. The experimenter then pointed to the stimulus card and said: "Remember this? Point to the one that goes with this." If the subject made an error, this procedure was repeated three times. If the subject still failed to respond properly, he or she was dropped from the study. The last step in the sample trial required the subject to tell the experimenter how to play the game. This latter step was to ensure that the subject was exposed to four pairs of completely different pictures. Instructions accompanying each pair were: "See these? This one goes with this one. Remember the trick. These are the same. Same things go together." Each pair was exposed for 5 s. Then, a response array card containing nine items was displayed before the subject. Stimulus items were presented in random order, and the subject was asked to point to the correct response picture. This procedure of viewing the pairs, hearing the accompanying instructions, and then selecting correct responses from the response array card was repeated until the subject completed three trials with 100% accuracy. If this did not happen within 10 trials, the subject would have been dropped from the study. No subjects were in fact dropped.

The sample trial for the sentential condition was essentially the same as in the above-described similarities condition. This time, however, the trick was described as follows: "These go together . . . we can put them together in a sentence. Now remember the _____ (point to the top picture) is on the _____ (point to the bottom picture)." This was followed by four new pairs of pictures under the same conditions described previously.

For rehearsal training, the procedure was equivalent except for the new trick, which the experimenter described as follows: "This one has a name, that is, box (point to the bottom picture). This one has a name, that is, star (point to the top picture). It helps to say the names again and again."

The posttest employed a paired-associate format similar to that used in the strategy-training phase of the study. Following retraining on each of two strategies, subjects were posttested.

The posttest used a set of 12 pairs of pictures. Again, each pair of pictures was selected to appeal best to one of the three strategies in the study. Four pairs were included for each of the three strategies. Pictures in the posttest were novel (i.e., not those used in the training sessions). Thus, the posttest comprised a near transfer task for all subjects on the two types of pairs for which they had been trained. In addition, each subject was given the third set of materials (i.e., those designed to elicit the strategy for which he or she had not been trained). This "transfer task" was designed to test further generalization and task-adaptive behavior.

The pairs were presented in a random order for 5 s each. No instructions for use of a strategy were given. Again the subject was asked to view all the pairs, then to view each of the stimulus pictures and pick the correctly associated picture from a card displaying an array of all response possibilities. The experimenter recorded the number of trials to criterion (100% correct, 1 time) to learn the 12-pair set and the number of errors within each strategy category.

Because assessing whether the subject was actually using the trained strategies or learning the pairs in some other way was a major problem for the study, a posttest interview was included. The interview attempted to identify whether the subject was aware of the strategies used, which were used, and, along the dimension of easy/hard, how they were perceived. Unfortunately, our subjects were completely unable to give us any insight into their strategy usage. This, in part, led us to the design of studies that placed children in peer groups and asked them to talk with each other. The rationale for this methodology is discussed further in Chapter 4.

The measure of performance on the transfer task was designed to indicate the effectiveness of strategy training. Scores were reported as the trials to criterion on the untrained set of stimuli. Mean trials to criterion revealed a tendency for the learning-disabled group to be more efficient (trials to criterion = 2.43) than the other two (nonhandicapped = 3.12, slow learning = 3.10). When transfer performance was measured as the number of errors made on the untrained task, the following mean scores resulted: learning disabled = 1.64; nonhandicapped = 4.04; slow learning = 2.90. An analysis of variance used to test group differences on these scores approached significance (F (2, 76) = 2.67, $p<$ .075). These are unusual findings in the light of previous research, which reports consistent difficulty in achieving transfer in mentally handicapped populations. In our study handicapped children did as well, if not slightly better, than their nonhandicapped peers.

These results can be viewed as relatively strong performance for the handicapped groups or as relatively weak performance for the nonhandicapped. In fact, both perspectives might be justified. MacMillan (1972) also reported superior performance on the part of handicapped children in a study of strategy training on a memory task. It is possible that the performance of the nonhandicapped groups in both studies was impeded by the imposition of unnatural or nonspontaneous strategies or, at least, an unnatural approach to strategy selection. The nonhandicapped groups, on the other hand, have been characterized by their tendency to fail to generate strategies (spontaneously) in an unprompted situation. For these children, dual-strategy training seems to be an effective means for stimulating the process of strategy usage, selection, or both.

The data reported thus far offer no direct evidence, however, that trained handicapped children were approaching the task strategically; that they were using those strategies actually trained; or that they were using strategies differentially based on either task demands or personal preference. There is some indirect evidence that does suggest specific effects of strategy training. Training in verbal mediation strategies on the sentential task seems to improve posttest performance generally and to decrease the number of errors on the transfer task significantly. It appears that those children who had more practice (trials to criterion) using verbal mediation strategies tended to remember more on a novel, subsequent task and to make fewer errors. Since children were exposed equally to two kinds of strategies in this study, the singular relationship between sentential strategy training and transfer-task performance indicates, albeit loosely, some selectivity in strategy usage.

Conclusion

Strategic behavior in learners with cognitive impairments is limited by a number of factors, including passivity; a tendency to remain at a fuzzy and imprecise level of concept or rule formation; and environmental circumstances that aggravate limitations. These impairments to effective strategic production seem to persist at all levels and in all aspects of processing. An attempt to train "good" strategies, those associated with effective learning in nonhandicapped populations, seems to define the problem too narrowly. It fails to account for differential preferences, abilities, and disabilities as well as for differential experiences and knowledge stores. In this chapter we have attempted to describe those kinds of strategic or not-so-strategic approaches that are more typical of cognitively impaired populations. Furthermore, we have attempted to provide evidence for the ability to perform at least some kinds of strategic or nearly strategic behavior in those populations. We suggest that these provide the optimal starting point for intervention.

4
Man Is the Measure of All Things

Our ability to observe spontaneous strategy usage or to instill effective strategies depends on how well we can observe them in their users. In this chapter we will focus on some of the methods that have been used to examine strategy use on a number of problem-solving and memory tasks in handicapped and non-handicapped populations. Some of these measurement techniques have been developed to tap well-known and successful learning strategies, both verbal and nonverbal, such as rehearsal and categorization. The most widely researched strategies have tended to be those that can be most satisfactorily measured. Nevertheless, numerous ingenious systems have been devised to overcome some of the measurement problems involved in accessing more elusive strategic behavior. We will describe some of these studies in detail and attempt to evaluate the degree of success with which they have achieved their goal. This brief survey does not presume to be a comprehensive review of all possible types of strategic behavior or measurement techniques. Our aim is to offer a sampling of various measurement possibilities, verbal and nonverbal, direct and indirect, covering a range of behaviors including memory, problem-solving, and academic skills.

Measurement of Strategy Usage

We will first examine some of the problems that cause difficulty in measuring learning and memory strategies, and some of the methods that have been developed to circumvent these difficulties. These have included direct observation of behavior, overt verbalization during performance, and obtaining verbal reports during or after the event. Most of these methods, including the first, have relied to some extent on verbalization, which is a problem for a number of reasons: it is difficult to observe, it is dependent on the verbal ability of the subject, and it relies on the accessibility of cognitive processes to introspection. The first two objections have been addressed by the development of nonverbal measures, including physical strategies such as sorting and categorizing (Salatas & Flavell, 1976), and pictorial techniques for measuring strategy awareness (Wellman, 1977). Of course, the first avoids rather than overcomes the problem, since it does not really provide a method of measuring verbal strategies. The need to develop a measurement device or devices sensitive to all forms of verbal and non-verbal strategic behavior is expressed well in the following passage:

Given the proper task and conditions of observation, one can often literally see and hear the older child's highly active and persistent attempts to store material for future retrieval; he may mouth or subvocalize item names over and over, physically cluster object pictures into groups by conceptual category, or otherwise show you that he has something more planful and future-oriented in mind than the mere perceptual identification of the items presented to him (Appel et al., 1972, p. 1366).

Direct Measures of Strategy Performance

The easiest strategies to observe in action are those manifested in overt behavior. The usual procedure is to pick a task that can be facilitated by the strategy under examination and to develop a method to elicit evidence that indicates whether this strategy has been employed. Some of the strategies that have been operationalized in this manner are categorization and manipulation of objects and pictures in memory research (Wolff & Levin, 1972) and problem-solving strategies such as scanning and focusing (Bruner, Goodnow, & Austin, 1956). Researchers have been quite creative in developing appropriate tasks; however, it is apparent that not all strategies can be operationalized in this way. Some tasks demand purely verbal strategies; in these cases, object manipulations, for example, might be merely imperfect reflections of these verbal strategies. Similarly, it would be foolish to assume that subjects who are not seen to employ the designated strategy are using no strategy at all or, in the case of an experimenter-imposed strategy, that subjects can necessarily make use of the experimenter's aid. Nevertheless, experimenter-imposed strategies, whether well suited to the learner or not, may have value beyond their observability since, as Borkowski, Levers, and Gruenenfleder (1976) have emphasized, the use of any active (frequently synonymous with overt) strategy may be important in ensuring transfer, especially for handicapped children. Comparison between the relative benefits of subject-generated strategies and experimenter-provided strategies has produced conflicting findings depending on the type of task and the age of children, as well as other factors (Flavell, 1970; McCarver, 1972).

Memory

McCarver (1972) investigated the effect of experimenter-imposed chunking on free recall in kindergarten, first-grade, fourth-grade, and college students. Pictures to be memorized were placed in a row either evenly spaced or divided into pairs by spatial and time groupings. Subjects in the chunking condition were also told that the best way to remember the pictures was to learn them in sets of two. Only the two older groups were able to make use of the chunking cues. Merely providing organization for the younger children did not improve their performance. Rosner (1971) has also found that chunking is an effective strategy for fifth but not first graders. Consider a hypothetical experiment that purported to measure the effectiveness of a chunking strategy, but used only young children as subjects. The conclusion that chunking is not an effective strategy for remembering a series of pictures would be tempting but unfounded, since merely presenting the pictures in chunks does not ensure that the children will be able to make use of this strategy. Many studies have, in fact, shown that chunking *is* an effective strategy for adults (Mayzner & Gabriel, 1963; Wickelgren, 1967). Nevertheless, when a child does not avail herself of a demonstrated strategy, the question remains as to whether there are age-appropriate or child-appropriate alternatives that would be more effective.

A related issue raised by this study is the fundamental question of whether young children even realize that something special must be done in order to memorize. To study this issue, Appel and co-workers (1972) carried out their study under two conditions, in only one of which were children told to remember. They found differences between first and fifth graders in their strategic behavior. They observed children presented with an array of pictures under "look" and "remember" conditions, noting study behaviors in 15-s periods. The behaviors recorded were sequential naming, sequential pointing, rehearsal, and categorization. Agreement between two observers varied from 0.89 to 0.97 on the four behaviors, suggesting that they could be measured reliably. The first graders appeared to use sequential naming as a strategy in the "remember" condition, but it did not improve their recall. Among the fifth graders, recall correlated positively with sequential naming and categorization and negatively with rehearsal, which seemed to interfere with categorization. In a second experiment, pictures were shown in sequence and naming, cumulative naming, and lip movement were recorded, with high reliabilities. Although strategy usage varied between ages and conditions, none of the behaviors were correlated with recall. The authors were puzzled by these findings and concluded that the children must have been employing effective study activities of *some* type, which were not externally observable. This study clearly demonstrates the impossibility of observing all that children are doing, even when selected behaviors are reliably recorded. In particular, the measurement of "lip movements" tells us nothing of what the children were saying to themselves. As the authors point out, "We would hardly want to claim that these 'tip-of-the-iceberg' observations really provided a clear, undistorted window into the Ss' mental actions vis-a-vis the items" (p. 1379).

The success of the first experiment by Appel and co-workers (1972) may have been due to the greater observability of the successful strategies, including categorization. A number of other researchers have used this technique to study memory performance. Torgesen and colleagues (1979) found large differences in the recall of learning-disabled and average fourth-grade children for an array of 24 pictures. However, after the children were given an orienting task in which they were asked to sort the pictures according to category, differences between the groups disappeared. The authors assume that the learning-disabled children were alerted to the categorical structure of the material, which aided recall;

unfortunately, they do not give evidence of sorting or clustering behavior on the recall task that would have reinforced this conclusion. A similar benefit from providing categorized pictures or prompting recall by category has been reported for mentally retarded children (Gerjuoy & Spitz, 1966). In this study, either presenting pictures by category or presenting them in random order but asking for recall by category (e.g., "Tell me about the *toys* you saw") succeeded in inducing equivalent recall in mentally retarded and average mental-age peers.

Tenney (1975) asked kindergarten, third-grade, and sixth-grade children to compose lists of words that would be easy to recall. By inspecting these lists for evidence of category organization, she was able to examine the students' awareness of the advantage of this strategy. The third and sixth graders used more categorical structure than controls and showed more clustering on recall when using their own organization than when the experimenter imposed a categorical structure on lists to be learned. The kindergartners, on the other hand, were unable to produce their own categorized lists, but benefitted from experimenter-imposed category structure.

Naturally, we cannot assume that Tenney's children would employ the categorization strategy if they were presented with lists to remember; we will see plenty of evidence that they do not necessarily do so. In a similar situation, Salatas and Flavell (1976) asked first graders whether categorizable or uncategorizable pictures are easier to remember, and whether a categorizable set is easier to remember if the pictures are grouped by category. Although children who had just had the experience of taking part in a memory task were more likely to answer correctly, there was no difference between those who had previously used categorization and those who had not. Even more striking was the fact that on retest, 6 weeks after the initial session, categorization was not predicted by correct answers to the two metamemory questions.

Cavanaugh and Borkowski (1980) studied categorization in kindergarten and in first-, third-, and fifth-grade children in two different tasks, free sort and cognitive cuing. In the first task, children were told to do anything they liked to remember a deck of 15 categorizable items. Six different study behaviors were observed with high interjudge agreement. The cognitive cuing task involved sorting a 30-item deck into 10 file boxes with cue pictures, the pictures remaining visible during recall. Both of these techniques enabled sorting strategies to be clearly seen and measured and revealed a developmental trend toward more categorical sorting and better recall. Consistent strategy use was not seen until the fifth grade. In addition, there was a significant developmental trend in the correlation between type of strategy and recall performance.* Strategy use also correlated with some aspects of metamemory (as measured by a questionnaire developed by Kreutzer, Leonard, & Flavell, 1975), with a few consistent rela-

---

*There has been some suggestion that mnemonic strategies evolve as a result of school-based environmental demands rather than as a natural course of development. Mnemonic strategies are not often observed in illiterate cultures or in children less than 8 years old (Brown, 1978).

tionships such as that between the study plan subtest of the questionnaire and fifth-grade strategy usage. However, unlike the direct-strategy measures, answers to the metamemory questionnaire did not predict performance on the memory tasks within grades.

Another strategy that has been investigated by observation of behavior is the use of physical manipulation to connect paired-associate objects (Wolff & Levin, 1972). Kindergarten and third-grade children who either observed the experimenter make the toys interact or did so themselves performed significantly better than control subjects. In the third grade, merely imagining that the two toys were playing together was equally facilitative. Improvement of performance was taken as a measure of effective strategy usage (imagery), and it was inferred that kindergarten-age children had limited ability to generate and use covert mental images. In a second experiment, children who manipulated objects that they could not see performed better than children who merely held the objects and tried to imagine them playing together. The authors add the interesting comment that "the attitude of Ss in the manipulate condition—head motionless, eyes turned 'inward'—suggested that they were actually experiencing mental images of their activity, and Ss subjective reports lend additional support to this conclusion" (Wolff & Levin, 1972, pp. 544–545). That the children were missing critical and typically visually provided information is likely to have had a positive effect on their use of strategies as well. Missing information serves the purpose of triggering more active processing in order to complete the image. This activity is itself associated with improved recall (Bransford, Franks, Morris, & Stein, 1979; Craik & Lockhart, 1972).

Maintenance of the active strategy of physical manipulation was tested in a similar paired-associate study, with the addition of a transfer task (Borkowski et al., 1976; Wanschura & Borkowski, 1975). Children were trained to place one object of the pair in, on, or under the other. During the posttest, no instructions to mediate were given, but unprompted manipulations were recorded. Not only were children who had learned the active strategy more likely to manipulate the objects during the transfer test, but they also tended to maintain their recall performance.

Moynahan (1978) compared first-, third-, and fifth-grade children's paired associate performance after they had been taught both an object interaction and a repetition (rehearsal) strategy. Stimuli consisted of small objects presented in pairs. The children were taught either to make the objects do something together or to say the names out loud over and over again. The authors were thus able to monitor the use of both strategies. Not only did they find the interaction strategy to be much more effective, but they also found that 80% of the children who said they had been more successful on the repetition task chose to use interaction on an untrained transfer task, compared with only 67% of the children who thought they had done better on the interaction task. This finding again demonstrates the unreliability of the verbal reports of these young children, who used neither strategy overtly on the transfer task, suggesting that several of them used one of the strategies covertly or used untrained strategies.

Problem Solving

Direct observation of problem-solving strategies has been used in a number of tasks with a similar format; the subject's task is to guess the correct one of a number of choices by a process of elimination. A variation of the 20-questions problem was developed by McKinney (1973) with the express purpose of observing strategic behavior directly. A child is shown pictures of 16 flowers that vary along four dimensions: size, color, number of petals, and shape of center. The task is to guess which flower the experimenter has in mind by asking "yes/no" questions. McKinney observed a developmental progression from random guessing among kindergartners to systematic scanning of specific flowers by slightly older children. The more efficient focusing strategy, in which half the flowers are eliminated by each question (e.g., "Is it red?") was rarely seen in children less than 9 years old.

A similar developmental sequence was seen in the Pattern Matching Task, also developed by McKinney and associates (Haskins & McKinney, 1976; McKinney & Haskins, 1980). Materials for this task consist of a problem board with eight designs, each composed of a circular arrangement of eight black and white dots in various combinations. A selected design is hidden, with each dot behind a movable shutter. The child may open shutters one at a time to determine which is the hidden pattern. As in the 20-questions problem, the most effective strategy (focusing) is that which eliminates half of the possibilities on each trial. The onset of some type of systematic strategy, in which a deliberate attempt was made to avoid noninformative moves, occurred around the age of 9 years, with optimal use of the focusing strategy becoming established at the age of 12 years.

In addition to the study of developmental trends in strategic behavior, this direct observation technique has application in the evaluation of individual differences such as cognitive tempo (McKinney & Haskins, 1980). While training in use of the focusing strategy improved the performance of impulsive children, instructions to slow down and think did not. This finding has profound implications for the modification of impulsive behavior, which may be best achieved through remediation of performance deficits rather than by attempting to alter the child's response style.

Academic Skills

Although most research studies of strategy usage have been carried out using problem-solving or memorization tasks, it is likely that most teaching of strategic behavior in the schools occurs in the context of direct instruction of academic skills. Some investigators have recently turned their attention to the experimental evaluation of educational strategies. An example is the area of reading comprehension, where an interesting method has been developed to study students' awareness of the importance of the various structural units contained in reading passages (Brown & Smiley, 1977). Children were asked to delete progressively more important sentences using different colored pencils, giving concrete evidence of their thought processes. Although all age groups showed a pattern of increased recall from the least to the most important units, only 18-year-olds were able to differentiate all four levels in their ratings. Eight-year-olds rated all four levels as equally important, whereas 10-year-olds were able to discriminate the most important and 12-year-olds the most and least important. Although this study appears to be an example of direct observation of strategy usage, it should be noted that the children were not necessarily using the technique to increase recall. The finding of increased recall for the more important units may simply mean that these sentences are easier to recall, and may not imply that the children were unconsciously assessing level of importance.

In the area of mathematics, Montague and Bos (1986) investigated the effect of strategy training on verbal math problem solving. Learning-disabled adolescents were taught an eight-step problem-solving strategy, each step requiring verbalization or a written response. The steps were as follows: (1) Read the problem aloud. (2) Paraphrase. (3) Visualize (draw a picture). (4) State the problem. (5) Hypothesize. (6) Estimate. (7) Calculate. (8) Self-check. Training was followed by a generalization test the following day and maintenance tests after 2 weeks and 3 months. All six subjects showed substantial improvement in performance, and four of the six reached the established criterion for generalization and maintenance. It was noted that the time taken to complete the tests increased substantially as a result of the training, but then decreased somewhat without an increase in errors. Fading of different strategy steps over time was evident for different subjects. The authors remark that the strategy was adapted to fit the individual needs of the problem solver. One major advantage of the method was that use of certain critical steps such as hypothesizing could be monitored and error sources detected.

Verbal Strategies

There are numerous examples in the literature of attempts to measure the spontaneous or trained use of such memory strategies as naming, rehearsal, and elaboration (Jensen & Rohwer, 1963; Taylor & Turnure, 1979). The difficulty of such measurement compared to that of overt nonverbal behavior such as sorting has been very evident, as we have seen in the study described in the previous section (Appel et al., 1972). Shepherd, Gelzheiser, and Solar (1984) attempted to measure both sorting and clustering and also the verbal strategies of rehearsal and self-testing in the free recall of classifiable pictures by learning-disabled and non-learning-disabled subjects. They found the first two strategies to be good predictors of recall, while the last two were not. However, as they point out, "it should be noted that the use of these strategies is difficult to observe reliably, and may in fact be occurring without being observed" (p. 9).

Various types of behavior were also observed in an experiment that was primarily concerned with the value of metacognitive awareness (Paris, Newman,

& McVey, 1982). Children were taught five alternative strategies for remembering lists of pictures—labeling, rehearsal, self-testing, physical sorting and clustering—and were then encouraged to choose any of these when performing the memory task. Study behavior was recorded by the experimenter, but unfortunately no information is given regarding reliability ratings of these observations. After training there was an increase in all strategic behaviors, which was only maintained in those children who had received an elaborated version of the strategy training in which a rationale was given for each strategy. Continued use of both the sorting and the labeling and rehearsal strategies contributed to improved recall scores; however, sorting behavior was primarily responsible for this increase. We can only speculate on the extent to which this finding may be influenced by the relative ease of measuring sorting behavior.

One of the easiest strategies to measure is verbal clustering on recall, which may or may not be related to category clustering during learning. This type of organization has been studied in children of widely varying ages and ability levels (Engle & Nagle, 1979; Robinson & Kingsley, 1977). Although most of these studies have found increases in recall with age and ability level, there has been conflicting evidence regarding changes in clustering with age (Glidden, Bilsky, & Pawelski, 1977; Robinson & Kingsley, 1977; Shapiro & Moely, 1971).

Engle and Nagle (1979) examined the effects of verbal elaboration training on free recall of categorizable objects. They found that semantic instruction increased both recall and verbal clustering. In a follow-up study, Engle, Nagle, and Dick (1980) investigated the ability of retarded children (chronological age 11 to 12 years) to generalize the elaboration strategy to different stimuli. Children were trained that the best way to remember a list was to think about each item in terms of its function, personal experiences, and its relationship to other items in the list. The importance of active involvement was emphasized throughout the first training day, but prompts were faded out during the second day. Semantic training on related lists resulted in improved recall and greatly increased clustering. This group also showed increased subjective organization, as measured by intertrial repetition of adjacent items; in other words, they imposed their own associations on the list. Posttesting with different lists 1 week later showed maintenance of clustering and subjective organization by the strategy training groups as well as better recall than the no-training groups. An interesting additional finding was that an equally strong and significant correlation between subjective organization and recall was shown by the strategy training and no-training groups. This reinforces the conclusion that lack of strategy implementation cannot be assumed in untrained control groups, and a more direct measure of strategy use is required. One attempt at this more direct measure was the inclusion of a post hoc interview in which subjects were asked how they had studied specific words. Responses were scored according to the extent to which they reflected use of the trained elaboration strategy. Unfortunately, there was no relationship between these ratings and either recall or organization scores or between trained and untrained groups. The authors conclude, "We interpret this as a failure of the interview technique and assume the oral self-report technique is insensitive to strategy usage" (Engle et al., 1980, p. 450). (See section on "The Adequacy of Verbal Reports" for further discussion of self-report interviews.)

Robinson and Kingsley (1977) found an equally strong relationship between clustering and recall in average and gifted second and fourth graders but noticed that, although the gifted second graders and average fourth graders showed equivalent levels of recall, the former showed much more sequential organization (i.e., more efficient retrieval). The authors also point out that the use of clustering as a recall strategy does not tell much about the cognitive strategies employed in producing it. A post hoc interview suggested that the older children, regardless of ability, used more sophisticated acquisition strategies than the younger children, in that they attempted to use some method of combining the words into groups. The difference in performance between average and gifted children was interpreted as evidence that the average children were able to formulate appropriate task strategies, but were less consistent about applying them.

The importance of differentiating between input and output measures has also been emphasized by Cavanaugh and Borkowski (1980) in a study of metamemory–memory connections on three tasks. In the first session, a metamemory questionnaire (Kreutzer et al., 1975) was administered to kindergarten and first-, third-, and fifth-grade children. Two weeks later, three memory tasks were administered. These consisted of free sort, in which children chose their own strategy for learning a categorizable list; cognitive cuing, in which the experimenter provided category pictures as cues; and alphabet search, in which letters of the alphabet were presented randomly and were followed by an unanticipated recall test. Clustering in retrieval was consistent for children in first grade and older; in other words, older children tended to use similar recall strategies across tasks. However, input strategy consistency did not appear until the fifth grade. An obvious problem with this conclusion was that measures of input strategy, although taken directly from observable behavior, may not have been as strictly comparable across tasks as the clustering measures. Results on the metamemory questionnaire showed that the older children were more aware of their memory than the younger children. Within each age group, however, verbalizable metamemory was not found to be necessary for successful performance.

Tenney (1975) also looked at both input (category structure) and output (clustering) measures in children's recall of word lists. She asked first, third, and sixth graders to compose lists of words that would be easy to recall. Some of the experimental groups were allowed to develop their own (self-directed) strategies, whereas others were guided in the use of a categoric structure as the basis for their lists. Strategies used were deduced from inspection of the lists. In general, the younger children did not use strategies in the recall conditions different from those used when they were free associating. They did, however, show more clustering and better performance on recall in the experimenter-imposed category condition than in the self-directed condition. The older children tended to use more categorical groupings when generating words for recall and more clustering in the self-directed condition. They also benefited from this strategy in the posttest. According to the author, inspection of the protocols revealed no evidence that children made strategic use of any type of relationship other than category structure.

Direct measures have also been employed to investigate verbal elaboration strategies. One widely used method to access input strategies is to ask children to verbalize their strategy aloud. Pressley, Levin, and Ghatala (1984) compared the keyword method with a naturalistic content method of learning vocabulary words. The content method required the child to compose a sentence in which the vocabulary word was used correctly. In the keyword condition, a keyword that sounded like the vocabulary word was given, and the child was instructed to make up a sentence containing the keyword and its meaning. An example was the word *casern*, meaning barracks. The chosen keyword was *case*, and the subject was encouraged to write a sentence including the words *case* and *barracks*. The sentence version of the keyword method was used specifically so that the authors could ask children to say the sentence they were using aloud, thus verifying that they were applying the desired strategy. The authors found that keyword recall was significantly superior to content recall. However, even children who said that the keyword method was better only used that strategy at better than chance levels when feedback or a prompt was included.

Glidden and her associates (Glidden, Bilsky, Mar, Judd, & Warner, 1983; Glidden & Warner, 1983) explored the use of verbal elaboration by educable mentally retarded adolescents in a free recall task. Subjects were trained to combine groups of words in experimenter-provided or self-generated stories. Recall was enhanced when the stories were provided or when the subjects generated their own stories from simultaneously presented blocks of words. When the words were presented sequentially, generating stories did not improve recall during training or transfer. Since strategy use was monitored during training, the authors were able to rate the stories generated on the basis of the number of words included and the level of connectivity. A significant correlation was found between story quality and level of recall. On the transfer trials, no instruction on the use of the trained strategy was given, and it was not possible to measure strategy usage directly. An indirect measure was obtained by analyzing study times under the various conditions. The authors concluded that most subjects were no longer performing the strategy, a conclusion that was supported by observation. In the concurrent condition, on the other hand, we are told that "all subjects mostly did what they had been told" (p. 98). It is not clear how this could be determined unless the subjects verbalized their stories aloud in this study.

Denney and Turner (1979) carried out a rather complicated experiment in which children performed four tasks: a signal task, in which the child was told to touch certain colored pages and not others; a match-to-standard task, in which the child selected the picture that exactly matched the standard from several distractors; a 20-questions task involving pictures of 20 common objects; and a paired–associate task using picture stimuli. Two different training conditions were applied, strategy modeling and strategy modeling with verbalization. In the first group, the experimenter performed the task with the child while explaining the appropriate strategy. The procedure was the same in the second group, except that the child was told to talk out loud while playing the game. The finding was that both experimental groups performed significantly better on the posttest than the control group, but that verbalization appeared to have no effect on performance. From our point of view there are two drawbacks to this experiment in regard to the way strategy use was measured. Typically, no attempt was made during posttest to ascertain whether children were employing the trained strategy. More interesting was the fact that, despite the purpose of the experiment—to explore the effects of overt self-verbalization—no record was made of the frequency and type of verbalizations (task relevant versus task irrelevant) during the posttest. We reiterate our original caution: in discussions of strategy measurement, examine carefully what is being measured and how.

Other studies of verbal mediation have not attempted to measure verbalization overtly, but have relied on improved recall as evidence of strategy implementation. A typical example is given by the paired-associate experiments of Milgram (1968), MacMillan (1972), and Gordon and Baumeister (1971). Milgram (1968) found no differences between normal and educable mentally retarded subjects on a series of lists involving experimenter-provided elaboration followed by self-generated elaboration, then by a reminder to mediate only. However, on follow-up a week later, the educable mentally retarded subjects failed to elaborate overtly and their performance declined significantly. MacMillan (1972) found that supplying mediating sentences during training was equally effective whether sentences were provided during testing or not. Gordon and Baumeister (1971) followed up MacMillan's study using a wider range of mental ages (6, 9, and 12 years). Subjects were either given sentences connecting pictures of objects or told to formulate their own sentences. Following training, strategy instructions were given on the first trial only. Both experimenter- and subject-provided elaboration groups of all mental ages learned the list more quickly and with fewer errors than the control group, although this effect was less marked for the groups of lower mental age. Although measures of response latency were taken, only total response times are given and are interpreted as evidence that additional time required to recall the mediator was outweighed by the increase in efficiency of learning. Individual response latencies could have provided an additional source of evidence that the elaboration strategy was being employed, as we shall see in the next section.

Indirect Methods of Measurement

A number of experimenters have used timing devices to infer certain types of strategy use, verifying their assumptions by developing hypotheses and setting up experiments to test these hypothesized patterns of time management. An example of this technique is the study of Glidden and co-workers (1983) discussed previously. The predicted pattern for the Story condition was that study times would increase for each item in a block as successive items were included in the story. Study time was also expected to be longer in the Question condition than for controls, but without any increase over the blocks. Although this pattern was indeed shown during training, differences were significantly curtailed during transfer. Since few subjects continued to use overt strategies during the transfer trials, the study-time data were interpreted as showing that they were not using covert strategies either.

Elaboration time was also employed in a study of visual imagery by Bugelski, Kidd, and Segmen (1968) using the peg-word method to instruct the meaning of lists of words. The method involved teaching the rhyme "one–bun, two–shoe ... " to college students. Subjects were then told to imagine the first peg word (bun) interacting with the first word on the list, and so on. Three interstimulus intervals were used (2, 4, and 8 s), only the last of which allowed sufficient time to create a satisfactory image. At the longest interstimulus interval, experimental subjects showed almost perfect recall, 30 to 40% better than control subjects. The absence of an experimental effect with the shortest interval, with an emerging advantage for the experimental group in the intermediate interval, provided strong evidence of some form of elaboration activity during the longer intervals, though not, of course, of the nature of that activity.

A similar use of time measurements was made by Belmont and Butterfield (1971), though in this case study time was taken to indicate rehearsal in a serial learning task. Retarded and normal subjects paced their own viewing of six-letter lists, each followed by a one-letter probe. Study times were expected to increase, at least for the first part of the list, to allow for cumulative rehearsal. A "fast finish" would indicate an attempt to hold the last few items in a short-term buffer. What happened was that study times of the nonretarded subjects increased throughout the list, and they showed strong primacy and recency effects on recall. By contrast, the retarded subjects studied each letter after the second for progressively shorter times, ending with a fast finish. The primacy effect was absent in recall.

In a second part of this experiment, Belmont and Butterfield (1971) forced subjects to pause on the fourth letter with instructions to rehearse the first four letters aloud three times. Another group were told to say each letter once and pass directly to the next. This was intended to prevent the subjects from rehearsing at all. Pause-time curves showed that the instructions were followed accurately. The effect on recall was enhanced primacy for the retardates in the rehearsal condition and reduced primacy for the normal group in the passive naming condition. Although these results show the usefulness of pause-time measures as indications of covert rehearsal, the authors point out that the rehearsal instructions did not bring primacy in the retardates up to the level of the normal group. They observed that normal subjects often used their eyes and fingers as an aid to memorizing and that rehearsal instructions did not translate exactly what was being done during the pause time.

Kramer and Engle (1981) used the pause-time measure with a group of average and retarded (mental age, 8 years) children in an attempt to measure near and far transfer of a rehearsal strategy. Groups of children were given the rehearsal training, strategy awareness training, or both, using free recall of pictures, letters, and numbers. Training was also generalized to telephone numbers, colors, and a list of grocery items. The rehearsal training consisted of teaching the children to pause after every fourth item and repeat the chunk three times. Two generalization tests were used to measure near transfer (recognition) and far transfer (serial probe). In addition to the recall measure, strategy application was assessed by self-paced exposure durations. On the maintenance posttests, rehearsal training was found to improve performance, and subjects who had received rehearsal training showed longer pause times at every fourth serial position. On the recognition transfer test, rehearsal training also resulted in longer pauses in these positions, especially when accompanied by strategy awareness training. No difference in performance was seen, however, probably because of ceiling effects. Effects of the training were not seen on the serial probe test, although there was a tendency for all subjects to spend more time studying the fourth item.

At the end of the final session, subjects were given a metamemory questionnaire to evaluate their awareness of the value of the memory strategies involved in these tasks. Although the strategy awareness training did result in higher metamemory scores, there was no relationship between metamemory and strategy usage or recall score, providing further evidence that metamemory questionnaires do not provide a good measure of strategy application.

The Adequacy of Verbal Reports

In creative problem solving as in memory tasks, subjects often are not aware of the stimulus that prompted their solution or successful recall, even when a hint is offered by the experimenter (Maier, 1931). This is true not only for experimental subjects but also for well-known artists and scientists, whose greatest discoveries often seem to have emerged from a flash of inspiration at a time when nothing was further from their mind. Asked what prompted the solution, they frequently insist that the idea just sprang into consciousness (Ghiselin, 1952).

One of the most common methods of eliciting information about thought processes is by obtaining verbal reports or introspections. Sometimes subjects are asked to "talk through" a thinking problem; on other occasions they report on the process after the problem is completed. Other investigators have posed hypothetical problems in which subjects describe their anticipated responses. A number of objections to these procedures have been suggested. Referring to research on basic memorial processes and encoding of perceptual information, Miller (1962) maintains that we cannot be aware of our mental processes, only of the results or products of those processes. Mandler (1975) states that many processes that occur at the unconscious level, including systems that analyze features of the environment and make affective appraisals, cannot be brought into consciousness. This view is supported by the failure of efforts to explain processes such as judgment of distance or pitch. More recently, this issue has been discussed in terms of implicit versus explicit qualities of thought processes (Johnson-Laird, 1983).

Although people show little conscious awareness of or ability to explain their perceptual processes, they are usually only too willing to give reasons for judgments and opinions or to describe their thought processes. Consequently, experimenters have continued to accept the premise that these introspections are valid indicators of the processes underlying complex high-level functions such as judgment, choice, and problem solving. Nisbett and Wilson (1977) have questioned the validity of these reports, arguing that subjective reports are so inaccurate as to be useless. Reports are based not on an awareness of cognitive processes that mediate a connection between stimulus and response, but on implicit theories about the plausibility or probability of such a connection. In other words, people respond to expectation, not awareness.

Nisbett and Wilson (1977) point out that studies attempting to manipulate subjects' responses have shown that subjects are frequently unaware that these responses have in fact occurred (Snyder, Schulz, & Jones, 1974; Storms & Nisbett, 1970). Alternatively, they may be aware of the response, but not that it represents a change from their initial position (Bem & McConnell, 1970; Goethals & Reckman, 1973). Subjects interviewed following an attribution experiment by Nisbett and Schachter (1966) were not only unaware of the experimental manipulation of their attributions, but proved to be extremely resistant to explanations of what had occurred. Although the deception often practiced in these studies casts some doubt on the validity of generalizing the results to everyday life, Nisbett and Wilson (1977) have attempted to broaden the base for their conclusions by carrying out a series of more naturalistic experiments. These experiments have been criticized on a number of grounds, both theoretical and statistical (Ericsson & Simon, 1980; Smith & Miller, 1978).

Subjects in one study, asked to compare the quality of four identical pairs of nylon stockings, showed strong positional effects favoring the right-hand pair. When asked to give reasons for their choices, however, they all insisted that their decisions were based on the quality of the stockings and denied the influence of position. As Smith and Miller (1978) have pointed out, as far as the subjects were concerned, the position of the stocking could hardly be viewed as the "cause" of their choice. From their point of view, the choice was made on the basis of quality comparisons, which happened to be made in a left-to-right order, each stocking being chosen if it was at least as good as the previous one. In another experiment, memorized word pairs were found to influence subsequent word associations, although subjects were unaware of this influence and gave other reasons for their choices. Again, the conclusions that subjects do not have access to their mental processes was based on their lack of awareness of a deliberately concealed experimental manipulation. Smith and Miller also object to Nisbett and Wilson's use of group-based statistical tests, which conceal the relationship between individual ratings and behavior. Reanalysis of the data from several experiments (e.g., Nisbett & Bellows, 1977) reversed the conclusions about the accuracy of subjects' reporting.

Ericsson and Simon (1980) have examined the findings of Nisbett and Wilson in terms of their own model and found general agreement, arguing that the vast majority of the results support the validity of verbal reports. In a thorough review of the literature, they give convincing evidence that verbal reports, "elicited with care and interpreted with full understanding of the circumstances under which they were obtained, are a valuable and thoroughly reliable source of information about cognitive processes" (p. 247). Situations favorable to obtaining valid reports include those in which the additional cognitive load imposed by the instruction to verbalize concurrently is negligible, in which the information is reproduced in the form in which it was acquired from the central processor without need for intermediate recoding into a verbal code, and in which information requested retrospectively concerns specific events rather then general interpretations. The requirement that verbal report shall not tax cognitive capacity is virtually impossible to meet in the study of young children and less so in the study of handicapped populations. In addition, accuracy will be greater if information is sought immediately after processing, when cues are still available in short-term memory. Processes that have been practiced to the point of automaticity will be resistant to verbal reporting.

Some of the evidence that has been cited as demonstrating the unreliability of verbal reports clearly violates these conditions. For example, Ericsson and Simon (1980) point out that investigations of creative insights rely on retrospective reports, which are often obtained long after the event. They suggest that these "sudden" insights are, in fact, the product of a gradual sequence of processes inaccessible to retrospective report. "Thinking aloud" protocols of problem solving have shown a clear sequence of background steps leading to these insights (Durkin, 1937). Ericcson and Simon also object to Nisbett and Wilson's (1977) use of between-subjects designs, questioning how subjects can be expected to remember the process by which they behaved differently from subjects in another experimental condition when their mental processes have never included such a comparison. In other cases, retrospective reports were obtained in which questions were phrased in such a way that it was not even clear that subjects were being asked to access information in long-term memory rather than to speculate about possible reasons for their behavior.

Smith and Miller (1978) discuss another important issue: the extent to which verbal self-report is a sufficient measure of access to mental processes. Evidence from many areas of investigation has shown that we can know more than we can tell. We may not be able to express this knowledge for a number of reasons, including difficulty in putting our thoughts into words, the failure of the experimenter to ask the right questions, and external factors such as social pressures. In addition, many processes are practiced to the point of automaticity when they become hard to access. Tasks most likely to be accessible to introspection are those that are novel and engaging and in which the report occurs close in time to the process.

Verbal Reports as Measures of Strategy Usage

The previous section provides considerable evidence that people are not necessarily aware of the reasons for their actions or able to report accurately on their mental processes. In discussing strategic behavior, we have quoted a number of experiments in which a discrepancy exists between measured use of strategies and subjects' reports of that use (Engle, Nagle, & Dick, 1980). A large number of studies also exist where self-report was the sole measure of strategy, which may have been "verified" by improved task performance.

The series of experiments by Shepherd and colleagues (1984) discussed previously included a paired–associate task, after which children were asked to describe the way they had studied. Data on the use of elaboration strategies taken from these reports led to the conclusion that learning-disabled and younger children were less likely to use elaboration than average and older children. There was also a good correlation between elaboration and recall in all groups. Unfortunately, details concerning these elaborations are not given.

Waters (1982) obtained retrospective reports from subjects of varied ages on the strategies they has used in a paired–associate memory task. Waters asked eighth and tenth graders which of four possible strategies they had used for each word pair memorized in a paired–associate task: reading carefully, rehearsing over and over, using visual imagery, and producing a verbal elaboration that connected the two words. The second two were combined as a measure of elaborative strategies. Subjects were also asked which strategy would have the best effect on recall. Metamemory was found to be significantly greater for subjects who had performed the task than for a control group asked to judge a hypothetical situation. Those who mentioned an elaborative strategy on the metamemory question were also significantly more likely to report use of such a strategy on the memory task, and to perform significantly better on recall. The more pairs elaborated, the better the performance. Although the author feels that these results provide strong evidence for the validity of verbal reports, it is not impossible that students who reported more use of elaborative strategies did so on the basis that they knew these to be valuable. That the more successful students should also be those with more highly developed metamemorial knowledge is also probable. These results are, therefore, suggestive rather than conclusive regarding the actual use of the reported strategies.

An additional finding of the Waters (1982) study was that tenth graders who reported elaboration were more likely to remember a word pair than eighth graders. This was interpreted as evidence that use of elaborative strategies was more effective in tenth graders. Since no report is given of actual strategies used, we cannot evaluate these elaborations in terms of effectiveness.

Visual imagery have been advocated as a mnemonic strategy (Paivio, 1971), especially for concrete nouns for which images are easily formed. Imagery is extremely difficult to access, however, and this can probably only be done by asking subjects to verbalize their images, which confounds the visual and verbal aspects of the strategy, or report on strategic behavior after the posttest.

An example of a post hoc report indicating the effectiveness of visual imagery is given by an experiment in which Bugelski and colleagues (1968) induced almost perfect recall of lists of words by teaching the peg-word method to college students. Subjects learned the rhyme "one–bun, two–shoe . . ." and then practiced forming visual images involving a bun and the first word on each list, a shoe and the second word, and so on. Not only did this result in impressive recall, even when several lists were learned in succession, but subjects were able to report vivid and unique image patterns for each pair.

Elliott and Gentile (1986) applied the same method to learning-disabled and nondisabled junior high school students and also produced a significant increase in recall for both groups, which was partially sustained over a 5-month period. Use of the strategy was evaluated by asking subjects to write down the images formed on the first list. This was not done for the other three lists, and strategy implementation was assumed on the basis of improved recall. Visual imagery has also been widely used in studies of paired–associate memory (Mondavi & Battig, 1973; Paivio & Foth, 1970; Yuille & Paivio, 1978). In some of these studies, subjects have been instructed in producing images (Jordan, Ackerman, & Wicker, 1977); in others, imaging has been inferred on the basis of the nature of the stimuli or assessed by posttest report (Mondavi & Battig, 1973). In the latter study, subjects were instructed to write down next to each pair what they had thought of when they were trying to learn that pair. Responses were classified into six categories: imagery, sentences, association or meaning, repetition, other (e.g., sound), and nothing. Imagery predominated for concrete pairs, but was hardly ever used for abstract pairs. However, imagery was much more strongly correlated with performance on the abstract than on the concrete pairs; in other words, subjects who were able to form images for the abstract pairs derived great benefit from this strategy.

Post hoc written report of strategic behavior was also used in a study comparing experimenter-provided visual mediators (PVM) with self-produced images (Jordan et al., 1977). The PVM subjects were provided with pictures that helped to relate the two words of a pair. Subjects in the visual imagery group were told to form a mental picture to help relate the two pictures. After the test, subjects were told to estimate the percentage of time spent using each of four methods of remembering the pairs: verbal association, common element, imagery, and repetition. The main finding of the study was that recall was almost identical for concrete stimulus pairs, but higher for abstract pairs in the PVM subjects. Experimenter-provided mediators were superior for stimuli for which subjects were unable to generate satisfactory images. Reported use of imagery was more frequent in both groups than any other strategy, but was much higher in the PVM group than in the visual imagery group.

A problem with this, as with all imagery studies, is that no check could be made of the actual use of visual images, beyond verbal report. That recall was superior for the PVM group on the hard-to-visualize pairs offers some support for the written reports indicating more imagery by these subjects.

Cavanaugh and Borkowski (1980) examined the connections between metamemory (i.e., reported understanding of the applicability of mnemonic strategies) and the actual use of those strategies. They used the entire interview developed by Kreutzer, Leonard, and Flavell (1975) to assess the metamemorial knowledge of first-, third-, and fifth-grade children engaged in three related memory tasks. Although a network of moderate intercorrelations between various metamemory and strategy variables was obtained, no predictable pattern based on those aspects of memory knowledge most closely tied to the tasks was found. In addition, there were no systematic differences in memory performance between children with high and low metamemorial knowledge, either broad or task specific. In other words, children's performance on the memory tasks could not be predicted from their answers to the metamemory questionnaires.

The studies cited above have all attempted to related reported strategy use to experimental behavior. Harris (1980) used interviews to examine "real-life" memory aids. Students and housewives were asked to rate how often they used each of a series of external (e.g., shopping list or calendar) and internal memory aids. The latter included such items as rhymes, stories, and verbal elaborations such as the key-word method. Subjects were also given a list of hypothetical events and asked how they would set about remembering and whether they would be successful. Very few of the internal aids were reported to be in frequent use, especially those that needed an encoding as well as a retrieval strategy. Harris (1980) points out that many of these strategies are so common that they are not thought of as aids but as "normal remembering," for example, clustering of categorical lists such a shopping lists. Others were mentioned in the open-ended questions but were not asked for specifically, so their frequency could not be estimated. In general, there was good agreement between the frequency with which aids were reported and the ways subjects thought they would go about remembering specific items or events. However, since no attempt was made to check the subjects' ratings of their ability to remember, the efficiency of their reported strategies could not be assessed.

In our own efforts to access strategy usage through interview procedures, we have met with unqualified discouragement. This was true whether our subjects were second-grade average, mentally retarded, learning-disabled, or gifted children or college-level average, learning-disabled, or low-achieving young adults. In most cases our subjects were at a loss for words. They simply stated that they did not know what they did. In the case of a charming but unhelpful gifted 6-year-old, she offered the explanation that the ideas simply popped into her brain.

At the college level we attempted to be more clever and to ask subjects to describe how they would advise a friend to attack a similar problem. We were met with overly general forms of advice such as to proceed carefully, think before you get started, and the like.

Group Setting as a Medium for Observing Strategic Behavior

Since it is so difficult to rely on subject reports, midtask verbalizations, or observations of nonverbal behavior, we have shifted our attention to observing children as they discuss strategy selections among themselves. This approach is motivated by methodological considerations as well as by some of the precepts of social cognition.

Methodologically, a group learning environment obviates the need for introspective, conscious self-report. The examiner has the opportunity to observe children in a seminaturalistic setting. If the charge is to work as a team and decide upon the best way to remember something, the observer becomes privy to the child's strategy selection process as he or she presents them to the group.

The social cognition literature suggests that social intelligence exceeds academic intelligence (Ames & Murray, 1982; Bearison, 1982; Berndt, 1981; Zimmerman & Blom, 1983). The group dynamic sets up a situation in which individuals confront immediate conflict about their ideas. The need for resolving the conflict requires reconsideration of the original thought, perhaps a clearer or more defended restatement of it, reformulations, or a novel approach. In any case, the group is likely to initiate deeper and more active processing. The group setting is likely, then, to increase the amount and the quality of discussion about strategy selection.

Conclusion

A number of conclusions can be drawn from the evidence presented in this chapter regarding the validity of various approaches to the problem of strategy measurement. In general, the more direct the measurement, the more accurately the strategy is represented. However, not all strategic behavior is accessible to direct measurement, and the attempt to translate verbal into equivalent nonverbal behaviors, for example, to allow more direct observation, is a partial solution at best. In fact, apart from concurrent verbalization, which is not always possible, no real impact has been made on the measurement of verbal strategies. Claims for the accuracy of post hoc reports are open to serious question.

The social cognition approach, touched on in the final section and discussed further in Chapter 5, has proved to be a novel and productive way to measure verbal behavior directly. A valid criticism of this method is that it can only respond to verbal behavior of individuals in a group, which differs in several ways from that of individuals facing a problem on their own. With this constraint in mind, we nevertheless feel that verbal strategies produced in a group setting have some value as an indication of individual behavior and, in any case, are of considerable interest in their own right. In Chapter 6, we will describe in detail our research into the spontaneous mnemonic strategies produced by handicapped and nonhandicapped children in small problem-solving groups.

5
No Man Is an Island . . .

In our review of strategic behavior as well as in discussing the importance of error production in the development of cognition, we have touched on the topic that will be the major focus of this chapter. It has become clear that cognitive processes do not develop in a vacuum, but evolve, starting in infancy, through interaction with both physical and social environments. The infant explores with all senses, gaining knowledge of the physical world and, to some extent, acquiring cognitive skills. The failure of an environment lacking in human contacts to provide for the complete development of human potential is seen in the extreme cases of children brought up in isolation or by animals, such as Kamala the wolf-girl (Gesell, 1940).

Social cognition is a term that has been increasingly seen in the literature and is described by Damon (1979) as a "hot topic." This phrase is not applied exclusively to social knowledge (as distinct from physical knowledge), but has been extended to include the social development of all knowledge (Bearison, 1982). Many of those writing on early childhood development have produced concepts that are variations on the idea of social cognition: shared meaning (Kaye, 1982a, 1982b), collaborative cognition (DeLoache, 1980), external executive function (Bruner, 1973), mediated learning (Feuerstein, 1979, 1980), and others. Social cognition is an interactive process, the adult (initially the parent) responding to cues from the child, and vice versa. Not only do parents possess knowledge and experience to be communicated to the child, they also act as a monitoring device, providing the executive function (organizing, planning, checking) that will eventually be internalized by the child. This role is later adopted by an expanded group of "significant others": relatives, teachers, siblings, peers, and so on.

Our goal in the remainder of this chapter is to explore in greater depth the effects of some of these social interactions on the evolution of cognitive development. We will look first at the part played by adults, as guides and teachers, and then consider the effects of peer interactions in tutoring and group learning settings.

Evolution of Cognitive Processes Under Adult Guidance

The process of normal development involves interactions with adults, primarily mother (and father) and, later, teachers. Bruner (1973, 1985; Bruner, Olver, &

Greenfield, 1966) has described the coexistence of an (at least partly innate) acquisition process in the learner coupled with a support system in the social environment. The match between these two forces underlies the mechanism by which cultural knowledge is transmitted.

The effect of the social milieu on the development of thinking has been examined by those who have attempted to marry the approaches of psychology and anthropology to the study of culture and cognitive processes (Cole & Scribner, 1975). Cross-cultural studies have pointed out that knowledge can be transmitted informally, as part of daily activities, or formally, where there is intent to impart knowledge and skills or values and attitudes to the young (Cohen, 1971; Mead, 1934). Scribner and Cole (1973) distinguish between "capacities," such as remembering, generalizing, and forming concepts, and "skills," which refer to the ways in which capacities are utilized. Although capacities have been demonstrated in all cultural groups studied (Cole & Scribner, 1975), the development of skills is influenced by educational experience (Greenfield & Bruner, 1969; Luria, 1971).

Vygotsky (1962) drew a distinction between everyday and scientific "ways of knowing," mediated by informal and formal situations. In everyday life, knowledge grows from the bottom up as a result of a multitude of concrete experiences. These may never be formulated as a generalized concept or rule. Formal schooling operates from the top down, starting with a general rule and filling in the specific knowledge underlying this rule. As a result, those with some formal schooling tend to generalize learning from one problem to another, whereas unschooled populations often treat each problem as a new one (Scribner & Cole, 1973).

Another significant difference between informal and formal education is that the former relies to a large extent on observational learning, where the adult provides a demonstration of a skill that the child imitates, and there is little verbal formulation by either the model or the learner. By removing education from the social context of life, learning becomes an end in itself whereby information is exchanged almost exclusively through the medium of language rather than by example. Symbols become the objects of learning, separated from their referents in the child's experience. As we shall see, this can be the source of great difficulty for some children, who become designated learning disabled or mentally retarded.

A central feature of this discussion is the importance of social interaction in the evolution of higher psychological functions (Bales, 1950; Feuerstein, 1979; Piaget, 1950; Vygotsky, 1962, 1978). For these writers, problem solving with others is a necessary precondition for the development of individual thought and, perhaps more significantly, for the transmission of specific ways of thinking and learning.

Piaget described four stages of intellectual development. The first two are characterized by prelogical thinking, which is essentially egocentric. During the stage of *concrete operations*, which is usually reached at about 7 or 8 years of age, the child begins to develop cognitive structures that allow the assimilation of new information and the understanding of concepts such as conservation and reversibility. A whole body of experimentation has been carried out relating the acquisition of these concepts to participation in social interaction (Silverman & Geiringer, 1973). It has also been noted (De Meuron & Auerswald, 1969) that children from lower-class or slum families frequently do not reach the stage of concrete operations until the age of 10 years. This has been ascribed in part to the discontinuous communication style observed in these families, which leads to a delay in cognitive development.

One of Vygotsky's basic tenets (Vygotsky, 1978) was that development not only of knowledge but also of cognitive processes occurs first on the "interpsychological" (social) plane and later on the "intrapsychological" plane. Skills that children can only display in socially supported contexts are in the process of being learned and will later become internalized. The development of independent learning thus takes place within a framework of shifting control from the environment to the individual. Not only do cognitive skills emerge, but the awareness of and ability to manage cognitive functioning (metacognition) is taken over by the developing child (Wellman, 1985).

However, the ability to make use of a teacher's guidance varies tremendously within individuals, even those at the same stage of mental development. Vygotsky (1978) used the term *zone of proximal development* to describe the gap between "actual developmental level as determined by independent problem solving and the level of potential development as determined through problem solving under adult guidance or in collaboration with more capable peers" (p. 86). Those with a wide zone of proximal development will show greater potential for growth under guidance.

Day, French, and Hall (1985) have summarized the four mechanisms by which cognitive growth is transmitted, constrained, nurtured, and encouraged by the social world: (1) adults and older peers pass on knowledge and skills to children; (2) children can perform skills in social interactions that they are unable to use alone; (3) adults assume responsibility for other activities so that children can practice new skills; (4) adults withdraw support as children develop competence.

These concepts of social learning have far-reaching implications for understanding the processes by which information is communicated from "experts" (e.g., parents) to children in the early years. Hess and Shipman (1965) identified three types of behavior shown by mothers in helping their 4-year-old children solve different tasks. An "imperative–normative" style, in which instructions were given without explanation or justification, resulted in poor performance by the children. Mothers who used more elaborated styles and more differentiated language tended to have children who performed better and were more verbal. Since these studies focused primarily on group effects, no details are given regarding the actual interactions or their effect on the child's development of independent skills.

A longitudinal study was later conducted (Hess, Holloway, Dickson, & Price, 1984) that examined the relationship between maternal behavior and preschool abilities and followed up by assessing school readiness and sixth-grade achievement of the same children. Some of the maternal variables that correlated most highly with both school readiness and achievement at the age of 12 years were affective relationship between mother and child, efficiency of verbal communication, expectation for achievement, asking for verbal rather than nonverbal responses, invoking personal authority in disciplining (negatively), and belief in luck as a factor in success (negatively).

A more specific relationship between maternal and child behavior has been demonstrated in a study of mothers' memory demands and children's memory performance (Ratner, 1984). Mothers were observed in interaction with their 2½- or 3½-year-old children during four 2-h periods. All questions asked by the mothers were categorized as either event questions (e.g., "Where did you put your jacket?") or knowledge questions (e.g., "What does an airplane do?"). Memory performance was evaluated on two tasks, a production task (recall) and a verification task (recognition). No relation was found between memory demands and performance at 2 years, but for 3-year-olds event questions related to production and knowledge questions to verification performance. The author hypothesizes that event questions require the child to construct a representation that is not supported by external retrieval cues, whereas knowledge questions develop categorical knowledge by providing information about concept boundaries. In this way, different types of processing skills were developed according to the types of questions asked.

One series of studies has examined the specific interactions taking place during assisted problem solving of preschool children on a construction task (Wood, Bruner, & Ross, 1976; Wood & Middleton, 1975). The main purpose of the procedure was to examine the manner in which the child and adult (either the mother or an unknown tutor) interacted in achieving the goal of independent construction of the toy by the child. This process was described as "scaffolding." Initially, the child must be engaged in the task, which must be reduced to a size the learner can cope with. It was noted that children were able to recognize a correct solution before they were able to put together the steps required to construct it, and that they would not imitate actions whose purpose they did not comprehend.

The tutor acts as a director, keeping the child on task and moving him or her to the next step at the appropriate time, marking critical features and controlling frustration. These "executive functions," also known as *metacognition*, play a significant role in problem solving. The scaffolding is gradually withdrawn, but can be replaced at any time if the child indicates that he or she is not ready. The crucial step is the gradual transfer of executive control from the tutor to the child so that the child learns to monitor self-learning.

When the tutors were the children's mothers, the most interesting finding was that the most successful pairs were those in which the mother was responsive to the child's level of activity. The authors propose a *region of sensitivity to instruction* (akin to the *zone of proximal development*), which is defined as the level at which the child is asked to add one extra operation or decision to those already being performed. Mothers intervening within this region were also more responsive to feedback from the children, following the pattern of offering more help when the child failed and less help when the child succeeded. These two characteristics of an active, adaptive approach to the child's region of sensitivity to instruction resulted in a much higher level of successful construction by the children.

It may be worth pointing out that this approach necessitates allowing the child to make errors, so that the instructor can fine-tune the level of support. An error-free performance (guaranteed success) probably means that the child is not being pushed into the zone of proximal development. It has been suggested that vulnerable children are often protected from making errors by an overdirective environment (Stern & Hildebrandt, 1986), which fosters passivity and inhibits cognitive growth. On the other hand, the adult must be responsive to the child's indications of lack of understanding, offering increased support when the child is not ready to go it alone.

A number of other studies of the process by which young children learn under adult guidance have shown similar patterns of interaction (Gardner & Rogoff, 1982; Rogoff & Gardner, 1984; Wertsch, McNamee, Budwig, & McLane, 1980; Wertsch, Minick, & Arns, 1984). Wertsch and colleagues (1980) noticed changes in the mothers' level of support as the children became familiar with the demands of the task. In addition, parental regulation diminished with the age of the child.

Wertsch and colleagues (1984) point out the importance of considering the motives of adults in understanding their interactions with children. In many traditional societies, learning as a distinct activity, separate from productive or economic activity, does not exist. In their study of rural Brazilian mothers and teachers, Wertsch and colleagues (1984) found the mothers to be much more directive, allowing their children to carry out only those parts of the task they could perform effectively. The teachers, on the other hand, used indirect forms of regulation that required children to understand the strategic significance of their behavior. In this case, the teachers appeared to be concerned with the children's learning, the mothers with completion of the task. The concept of instruction within the child's region of sensitivity only makes sense when learning is viewed as an independent activity or goal.

For handicapped children also, the objective has frequently been that of correct performance rather than constant stretching of the zone of proximal development. Consequently, the emphasis has been on error-free learning within the realm of assumed capacity. Adults may also provide poor stimulation in deference to a child's cognitive shortcomings, to avoid making the child feel incompetent. Vygotsky complained about curricula that are based on the assumption that retarded children are incapable of abstract thinking, and advocated education aimed at the upper boundary of the zone of proximal development (i.e., that which can be achieved under most favorable circumstances):

Precisely because retarded children, when left to themselves, will never achieve well-elaborated forms of abstract thought, the school should make every effort to push them in that direction and to develop in them what is intrinsically lacking in their own development (Vygotsky, 1978, p. 89).

The concept of aiming instruction at the region just beyond the level at which the child is functioning has proved seminal in the recent development of educational programs for the handicapped (Brown & French, 1979; Feuerstein, 1979, 1980). Feuerstein (1979, 1980) has carried out much of his work with adolescents whose apparent retardation is rooted in early cultural deprivation. He emphasizes the importance of mediated learning experiences (MLE) in which adults continually question and extend the limits of knowledge of their children. In the absence of these opportunities, children enter school lacking in discourse skills, a situation exacerbated by their own and their teachers' perceptions of their inability to develop higher cognitive processes and a consequent emphasis on rote skills and concrete thinking. Feuerstein has developed two systems to assess potential and remediate early deprivation, the Learning Potential Assessment Device (LPAD) and Instrumental Enrichment (IE). He has successfully shown that many of those whose "retardation" is the result of a lack of MLE demonstrate a wide zone of proximal development, which can be traversed with appropriate intervention.

To be effective, mediators must not only give information, but must also help the child to interpret and organize and then to generalize experiences. In addition, children will become more aware of their cognitive processes and show an increase in metacognitive awareness. Much of the mediated learning that occurs on a daily basis is carried out by parents and may be incidental or intuitive, and not necessarily effective. A number of studies have shown that families of dyssocial children (especially "slum families") frequently show limited vocabulary and language usage, which has resulted in significantly retarded cognitive development in the children (Bernstein, 1962; John, 1963). Such children may perform like retarded children because they have lacked sufficient MLE.

Barriers to effective mediation may also be *created* by handicaps such as emotional disturbance or mental retardation in the child. According to Feuerstein (1980), intuitive approaches to mediation are less likely to be effective with handicapped children, and alternative methods must be developed. Like Vygotsky, Feuerstein argues against the tendency to educate these children by creating simplified learning environments (lacking in MLE) that assume an inability to cope with representation and symbolic thought or abstraction. On the contrary, by increasing the level of MLE, many apparently retarded performers can develop high levels of thinking. Feuerstein has developed a detailed and specific program of activities (IE) designed as a structure within which MLE can be provided. Numerous studies have been conducted in different countries and among various populations to investigate the effectiveness of the IE program. Results have varied according to circumstances, but it has been suggested that what is important is the mediational teaching style rather than the actual curriculum (Campione, Brown, & Ferrara, 1982).

This mediational style is part of the process by which an adult organizes the child's experiences to facilitate connection between two occurrences of the same object, word, activity, and the like, preparing children for the type of learning that takes place in school. Such structuring creates links between novel and

familiar problems, helping the child find similarities across contexts and allowing the child to apply his or her available skills and knowledge to new tasks
(Rogoff & Gardner, 1984). This process is facilitated by "headfitting," the regulation of the difficulty of tasks so that new information is compatible with existing
knowledge (Brown, 1979).

The role of the expert in helping children ("novices") transfer learning across
tasks is especially important for handicapped children, whose difficulty with
transfer and generalization is notorious. Stone and Wertsch (1984) have examined the interaction between a clinician and a learning-disabled child to determine how the process leads to improved cognitive functioning. The clinician
intervenes when the child fails to execute strategic aspects of the task correctly,
leading the child through the steps that caused the error in order to increase
awareness and provide the means to monitor errors. The skilled clinician does
not carry out the step completely, but aims to improve the child's ability to function independently. Changes in communicative patterns during the course of an
instructional session reflect a transition in the source of strategic responsibility
from the adult to the child. The child's task is to understand the definition of the
task situation that prompted the clinician's behavior, a type of metacognitive
knowledge important in generalization of the new skill. This so-called *proleptic
instruction* requires social inference that may be beyond the capabilities of a
learning-disabled child, because the specific processing difficulties of such children may interfere with these adult–child interactions. This may account for the
difficulties of learning-disabled children in developing self-regulative strategies.

An ongoing program by Brown and her colleagues (Brown & Ferrara, 1985;
Brown & French, 1979; Brown, Palincsar, & Armbruster, 1984) has investigated
the processes whereby a child is led to learn a new skill or concept, and the ability
of children to transfer this knowledge to new tasks both with and without further
training. Palincsar and Brown (1984) demonstrated the importance of aiming
interventions at the upper limit of competence, stretching this limit by moving in
small steps. Subjects were a group of children selected because of reading comprehension problems, for whom remediation had been limited to decoding skills
because of their supposed inability to comprehend. A tutorial dialogue, in which
the tutor modeled comprehension-fostering strategies and the child gradually
learned to play the role of leader, markedly increased both comprehension and
the ability to internalize the strategies necessary for independent learning. An
added advantage of this method was that teachers changed their opinions and
expectations of the child's capabilities. It is worth noting that the concept of
"upper limit" is not static; as the child progresses into the zone of proximal
development, the upper limit also advances.

A number of key concepts have developed out of the work of this group regarding the operational meaning of the zone of proximal development, the extent to
which the zone differentiates between different types of handicapped children
(e.g., mentally retarded and learning disabled), and the existence of different
dimensions of learning, including IQ, speed (measured by number of prompts
required), and breadth of transfer. In particular, Brown has emphasized the

importance of transfer in terms of reducing the number of prompts required in applying a new solution to a series of similar problems, a particularly troublesome area for handicapped children. It has also become evident that the zone is not unidimensional; although most low-IQ children are consistently slow learners and narrow transferrers, a significant minority have been found in whom various combinations of these dimensions coexist. For example, children may be fast learners and wide transferrers, fast learners and narrow transferrers (context bound), or slow learners and wide transferrers (reflective).

Brown and Ferrara (1985) proposed that learning-disabled children require less adult assistance than mildly mentally retarded children to master and transfer learning; in other words, they have a wider zone of proximal development. Findings by many researchers (e.g, Torgesen & Goldman, 1977) that, when given instruction, disabled learners can achieve as well as normal children give some support to this view. Hall and Day (1982) evaluated this proposal with retarded, learning-disabled, and normally achieving second-grade children, using a balance scale task in which children were given a series of increasingly explicit hints. They found the predicted differences only on transfer tasks, where the retarded children needed more prompts than the learning disabled for near transfer and especially for far transfer.

One advantage of using the zone of proximal development, rather than a static measure of IQ, is the implication that the zone can vary within different domains, depending on interest and knowledge as well as ability. It has been noted (Brown & French, 1979) that mild retardation is a "school disease," since retarded people are frequently able to learn nonacademic vocational skills and maintain themselves successfully in nonschool society. In other words, their zone of proximal development is much wider in nonacademic domains. It is also likely that the width of the zone will be especially variable for learning-disabled children, even within school-defined domains—an alternative way of approaching their oft-mentioned inconsistency.

Peer Tutoring

A special case of "expert–novice" interaction is that in which an older or more capable peer acts as tutor to a younger or less accomplished child. It has been suggested that this form of instruction may be as or more beneficial to the teacher as to the learner (McWhorter & Levy, 1971), either by encouraging some form of cognitive reconstruction or by modifying the self-concept and motivation of the tutor. Benefits from peer-tutoring arrangements have also been seen in settings where all students participate in turn as tutors and pupils. In this case, the effects have generally been ascribed to the increased "opportunity to respond" afforded by the peer-tutoring approach (Delquadri, Greenwood, Stretton, & Hall, 1983).

A number of studies have examined the ability of children to adjust their speech or their teaching to the age or ability level of their students (Ludeke & Hartup,

1983; Shatz & Gelman, 1973). Ludeke and Hartup (1983) found that 9- and 11-year-old girls used repetitions, strategic advice, progress checkups, direct assistance, and praise more frequently with younger than with same-age pupils. They concluded that the children had an implicit "theory of teaching" that assumed that younger children require both more cognitive structuring and more supportive feedback than same-age children.

The fine-tuning of instruction to the responses of the student described in the above example (Ludeke & Hartup, 1983) represents an ideal that is rarely achieved in regular classroom settings. A somewhat different approach involving classwide peer-tutoring systems, emphasizing quantity rather than quality, has been developed by Greenwood and his colleagues at the Juniper Gardens Children's Project in Kansas (Greenwood, Delquadri, & Hall, 1984). The stimulus underlying this approach was the finding that children in regular classrooms are rarely actively engaged in lessons. Observation of one fourth-grade child showed an increase in time spent in oral reading from an average of 10 s per day in the regular classroom to 6 min after he was placed in the learning-disabled classroom. A concomitant increase in reading speed and accuracy was seen after only 2 weeks.

The model developed by this group was designed to increase participation in classroom activities and focuses on behavioral response levels, rather than "cognitive development." The engagement of the child in oral reading, writing, and instructional interaction by providing systematic opportunities to respond is considered critical for academic achievement, especially for disadvantaged or learning-disabled children. Initially, the teacher explains the "game" and demonstrates the tutoring behavior, with ample opportunity for student involvement and corrective feedback from the teacher. On a daily basis, students work in pairs with the tutor offering feedback and awarding points; after 10 min the students exchange roles. The long-term goal is to enable more children to remain in the mainstream by increasing opportunities for active involvement in learning during the early grades. In an ongoing series of experiments, it has been shown that children can increase their academic behaviors from 20 to 70% during classwide peer tutoring. At the same time, a reduction in spelling and reading errors and improvements in oral reading rate, mathematics, and vocabulary have been demonstrated (Greenwood et al., 1984; Hall, Delquadri, Greenwood, & Thurston, 1982).

Use of the term *expert* suggests that the person most suited to the role of tutor will be the child who has mastered the information to be imparted. The studies just described suggest that this is not necessarily the case, that peers can act as tutors for each other, regardless of their level of achievement. The possibility that low-achieving children may also benefit from the tutorial role was investigated by Allen and Feldman (1973). The role of tutor was assigned to low-achieving fifth graders, who taught lessons in science, language, and reading to third-grade students. Before each lesson, the tutors were allowed to study the material to be taught and prepare for the lesson. On alternate days, tutors and pupils studied alone, thus acting as their own controls. It was found that over a 2-week period of five lessons and five independent study periods, the tutors' performance improved much more in the tutoring condition than when studying alone. The reverse was seen among the pupils. This latter finding may be understood in view of what we know about the optimal conditions for imparting knowledge. It is probable that low-achieving children are less successful than average children at monitoring the learning of other students, although case-study evidence of successful peer tutoring by low achievers is available (Steinberg & Cazden, 1979). Clearly, the effects on pupils must be taken into account, however beneficial the tutoring role may be for low achievers.

Possible reasons for the beneficial effects of the tutoring role are many. One explanation is that adopting the role of expert induces changes in role expectations resulting in an improvement in attitude and self-concept, especially among students who have experienced repeated failure. In addition, children may make more effort both to organize the material and to learn it thoroughly in order to be able to teach it to another—in other words, engage more actively in the learning process. It is also possible that interaction with another student during the teaching period may have increased learning, although this effect only occurred in conjunction with the tutors' original study period, since it was not seen among the pupils.

A number of studies have also examined the merits of tutoring for learning-disabled children, with generally positive results. Jenkins, Mayall, Peschka, and Henkins (1974) found that 7- to 10-year-old learning-disabled students tutored in word recognition, spelling, and multiplication by older, nonhandicapped students made greater gains than children in teacher-led small groups. Other studies have shown successful use of high-achieving sixth-grade students (King, 1982) or reading-disabled sixth graders (Lamport, 1982) as the tutors. In some cases, the pupils did as well as, but not better than, those in teacher-led groups (Kane & Alley, 1980; Sindelar, 1982).

Because of the number of variables involved (e.g., age and academic status of tutors and pupils, subject matter, length of intervention, presence or absence of control groups, nature of posttest), it is difficult to draw any firm conclusions about the most favorable applications of tutoring with learning-disabled students. In a recent review of relevant studies, Scruggs and Richter (1986) comment, " . . . It is difficult to imagine another instructional intervention in the field of learning disabilities which meets with such unqualified enthusiasm and, yet, is so lacking in empirical evidence" (p. 13). Interestingly, they agree that, in spite of the methodological challenges, "peer tutoring has great power and utility in special education" (p. 13).

Another group of exceptional children who have been found to benefit from peer tutoring are those with emotional or behavioral disorders. By teaching a younger, less able child, a student might be expected to gain in self-confidence as well as in academic knowledge. Benefits to both tutors and pupils have been achieved in studies where high school children classified as emotionally disturbed acted as tutors to elementary-age mildly retarded children (Maher, 1984). The program involved considerable training and support for the tutors, who worked with the pupils on arithmetic, reading, and language arts over a 10-week period. During this time, and during the follow-up period of one or two quarters, there was a significant increase not only in the academic performance of the pupils, but also in the assignments completed and test performance of the tutors; attendance also improved, and there was a reduction in disciplinary referrals. Tutors reported an increase in their awareness of the need to budget time for study and in their appreciation of the planning of their own teachers, a desire to improve their school performance, and a better outlook on their ability to succeed. Of the 16 tutors, 13 volunteered to continue the tutoring. No attempt was made to compare the benefits to the emotionally disturbed high school students from this program with those from some other intervention, such as counseling; however, that both tutors and pupils benefited makes this seem a cost-effective approach. The concept of using tutoring to create natural therapeutic environments in the classroom has also been discussed by Steinberg and Cazden (1979) in their case-study descriptions of peer teaching.

Studies in which behaviorally disordered students functioned as pupils rather than tutors have shown less favorable outcomes (Kreutzer, 1973). This is not altogether surprising, since the effects on attitudes and work habits assumed to underlie the benefits of acting as tutor would not occur. The existence of a general impact on self-concept and social functioning has also been questioned (Lazerson, 1980). In addition, it has been pointed out (Scruggs, Mastropieri, & Richter, 1985) that tutors are more likely to gain academic skills if they are somewhat deficient in the areas being tutored or if they need fluency-building activities.

Group Interaction

We have discussed at length some of the ways in which the social environment (in the guise of parents, teachers, and peers) interacts in a more or less purposeful way with the individual to promote cognitive growth by continually stretching the range of competence. Another perspective on learning within a social framework considers the impact on the child of working in small groups of children as peers, with similar learning goals.

Attempts to investigate social interaction effects in the classroom have resulted in numerous experiments on group or team learning (Sharan, 1980; Slavin, 1978). A number of interesting questions have been addressed by this research. Do high-ability children benefit only from interaction with children of similar ability, or can they gain from interaction with children less able than themselves? Do children of lower ability do better when grouped with more able children or with those of approximately the same capabilities? On a more practical level, what types of problems are likely to be encountered in working with mixed-ability groups, and what steps can be taken to minimize these difficulties? These questions are especially critical for those interested in creating optimal learning environments, in or out of the mainstream, for handicapped children.

It has for some time been common practice in the elementary classroom to divide children into small groups of comparable achievement for the purpose of instruction. It might appear that these groups would be characterized by coopera-tive endeavor. The usual pattern, however, is for the teacher to instruct one group while the remaining children read silently to themselves or work on other assign-ments. David and Roger Johnson and their colleagues have described three types of classroom interaction: controversy, concurrence seeking, and individualistic learning (Smith, Johnson, & Johnson, 1981). Of these, individualistic learning, in which children work alone without interaction and with independent goals, occupies 70% of classroom time (Johnson, 1979). Such learning as takes place in groups is likely to be of the concurrence-seeking variety, with emphasis on agree-ment and avoidance of arguments. This is not altogether surprising since, for many teachers (and students), controversy or conflict in the classroom implies lack of discipline and control. It should be noted here that the authors clearly view this type of controversy in a positive light as furthering both achievement and cognitive growth, as distinct from *competition*, which usually takes place in a setting that emphasizes individual learning.

One of the pioneers whose theory of cognitive development has been drawn on for the investigation of social interaction effects, especially those generated by conflict, is Jean Piaget (1950). According to Piaget, children less than 7 or 8 years of age show a primarily egocentric style of thinking in which processes tend to be static, concrete, and irreversible. From a Piagetian viewpoint, peer interaction helps break down a child's egocentrism, allowing "decentration" and the develop-ment of conceptual thinking during the period of concrete operations. A key Piagetian concept is that of "equilibration" or self-regulation, which can be fostered by the conflicts encountered during social interaction. These conflicts induce "cognitive restructuring" or the reformulation of ideas on the basis of information and arguments presented by other members of the group (Ames & Murray, 1982; Berndt, 1981). From this restructuring develops logical reason-ing, which is "an argument which we have with ourselves, and which reproduces internally the features of a real argument" (Piaget, 1928, p. 204). Johnson, Maruyama, Johnson, Nelson, and Skon (1981) agree that controversy promotes transition to higher stages of cognitive reasoning via greater understanding of another person's perspective.

The Piagetian model has formed the basis for numerous studies investigating the effects of social interaction on the acquisition of conservation, an operation that requires the reversibility of thought processes achieved as the child enters the stage of concrete operations. Silverman and Stone (1972) found that not only did nonconservers yield to conservers when working together on conservation-of-area problems, the effect was sustained on the posttest given after 1 month (using different configurations solvable by the same rule), and the nonconservers continued to give explanations provided by the conservers during the initial interactions. This was taken as evidence for generalization of the concept as a result of cognitive reorganization. Previous findings that conservation can be induced by verbal training without social interaction (Beilin, 1965) have failed to show generalization.

A series of studies using Piagetian tasks such as conservation and spatial perspective taking have been conducted by Doise and his colleagues (Doise, Mugny, & Perret-Clermont, 1976; Doise & Mugny, 1979; Mugny & Doise, 1978) and summarized by Perret-Clermont (1980). In these studies, it was shown that children working in pairs used more advanced problem solving than children working individually. Thus, children could often complete tasks when working with others that they could not manage in isolation (Doise et al., 1976). It was not necessary for the children to be exposed to the correct solution, but merely to experience a conflict of "centrations" requiring them to acknowledge and integrate a variety of perspectives. In other words, exposure to conflicting opinions was more effective in producing cognitive growth than simple communication, modeling, or imitation.

Our results indicate that, while collective exchange can certainly facilitate cognitive work and the formation of operations, *cognitive conflict in social situations*, in certain conditions, and at a particular stage in the development of the child, can actually bring this about directly (Perret-Clermont, 1980, p. 192; italics in original).

The experience of conflicting information alone may not be sufficient to stimulate cognitive growth. Perret-Clermont questions whether a child, faced with conflicting external data, would persist if working alone without "the incitement of social relations." In other words, *both* cognitive conflict and social interaction are necessary. The ability of people to ignore the evidence of contradictory information has been thoroughly documented (Wason, 1972; Johnson-Laird, 1983).

Like Feuerstein, Perret-Clermont focuses on the role of cultural deprivation, especially as it creates a gap between teacher expectations and the norms of the child's milieu, in creating apparent intellectual deficits. Perret-Clermont proposes that the type of teaching in which subject matter is presented simultaneously to all children (as in the typical United States classroom) does not take into account the needs of these children, which would be better addressed by encouragement of social interaction. She describes an experimental program carried out by Cecchini and his colleagues in Italy, which involved increasing the level of interaction and communication between the children, resulting in the elimination of linguistic deficits (Perret-Clermont, 1980).

We have already seen that in some circumstances cognitive conflict promotes intellectual growth (Piaget, 1950). A student encountering a different point of view begins to engage in active rehearsal of his or her own rationale and consideration of the opponent's position. This may also involve seeking further information with which to solve the conflict. The outcome of such an encounter may well vary, depending on the children involved as well as the specific learning environment.

Smith, Johnson, and Johnson (1981) compared the learning and attitudes of sixth-grade children in heterogeneous groups of high, low and middle ability, who had been instructed to engage in controversial discussion, with those of groups told to seek concurrence and with those of students studying alone. The authors found considerable advantages for the controversy groups in tests of subject matter given immediately after the study and again after 4 weeks. In addition, children in the controversy condition were more likely to seek additional information (where this involved time and effort), had more positive attitudes toward the subject matter and toward argumentation, and perceived more academic support from their peers. On most of these measures, concurrence-seeking groups took an intermediate position.

When the performance of high-, low-, and middle-ability children was examined separately, it was found that middle- and low-ability children in both group conditions achieved and retained more information than those in the individualistic condition. Apparently group discussion, even without conflict, eliminated some of the effects of ability, perhaps because of increased motivation, perhaps because of reduced reading requirements when much of the learning is produced by oral discussion. For the high-ability students, concurrence seeking was least effective. Johnson and colleagues (1981) described the effectiveness of cooperation, not only in increasing achievement, but in enhancing emotional involvement and motivation and reducing fear of failure. Presumably these benefits occur even without the controversial exchange of ideas and information and are more significant in promoting success for lower-ability students.

A study by Forman and Cazden (1985) examined the problem-solving behavior of pairs of children in terms of both Piagetian and Vygotskian concepts. Children were asked to cooperate in a series of chemical reaction problems in which the task was to determine, by a process of combinatorial reasoning, which chemical(s) caused the color change in a reagent. The three dyads in the study showed different patterns of interaction, with two developing a consistently cooperative format. By the later stages of the experiment, these pairs were also more likely to use deductive combinatorial strategies and to be more successful in producing the correct solution. However, this did not necessarily transfer to an individually administered posttest.

Forman and Cazden discuss the role of cognitive conflict (conceptualized as Piagetian) in problem solution for these dyads. The situation in which conflict most frequently arose was that in which children disagreed about the conclusions to be drawn from their experiments. They were then forced to reevaluate the evidence and either revise their conclusions or formulate a clear defense to convince their partner. However, this was only one of the mechanisms by which growth occurred; Forman and Cazden also describe a pattern of mutual guidance and support in these dyads that enabled them to solve problems they were unable to solve independently. This was seen as evidence that the children, aided by their peers, were working within their zone of proximal development (in other words, was supportive of a Vygotskian perspective). The process of deductive combinatorial reasoning was internalized immediately by some of the children; for others, this was seen in a delayed posttest. The dichotomy between Piaget's approach, based on conflict, and that of Vygotsky, based on supportive inter-action, may be a little simplistic; the subtleties of human interaction are almost certain to involve both forms of development.

Group learning can have two major objectives, group product and individual learning, which are by no means always served by the same variables. Where per-formance within the group is one of the goals, the task of getting the right answer as quickly as possible may preclude discussion of strategy and process. The problem of focusing on quick solutions rather than group interaction is especially evident in heterogeneous groups, where the most able children answer most of the questions. This may be a very efficient way of getting the job done, but proba-bly does not promote learning, especially in the nonresponders.

In an early example, the relative efficiency of heterogeneous groups in a task requiring members to make as many words as possible from the letters of a multi-syllabic word has been shown to depend largely on the most able member of the group (Watson, 1928). Even so, summing the output of the members working alone would be more productive. The author tested only total output, not individual learning, in the two conditions.

In looking at benefits to be gained by low-achieving children from group inter-action, therefore, we should consider gains in individual learning and cognitive skills rather than in group productivity. Although group interaction may promote accomplishment of an assigned task, lasting changes may only be possible if progress toward higher-quality reasoning is achieved during the cooperative effort. This was described by Forman and Cazden (1985) in the study of chemical reagents described above. Skon, Johnson, and Johnson (1981) found similar effects in a study of categorization and retrieval, in which first graders in a cooperative condition showed not only better recall, but also more use and aware-ness of the categorization search strategy than those in a competitive or individu-alistic condition. This was especially impressive since Salatas and Flavell (1976) found that even third graders had difficulty using a category search strategy when working individually.

In a study of the impact of group discussion on the development of abstract concepts, Kol'tsova (1978) examined the concept formation of ninth graders under group and individual conditions. In the group condition, students were given an assignment and encouraged to formulate a plan for carrying it out, exchanging opinions and discussing problems that arose. Afterward, students were tested individually on their understanding of the concept. In the control classes, students carried out the assignment independently and all communica-tion was forbidden. On the whole, group discussion proved an effective method of learning the concept. The clarification of ideas as a result of the critical evalua-tion of different views led to more rigorous definitions of the concept and a greater depth of generalization. Not only knowledge, but also methods for the most effective organization of knowledge were exchanged. Not all groups were equally successful, however, and the variation between the groups enabled the author to draw some conclusions about the variables leading to success. In general, groups in which all the members participated actively were most successful; the amount of experience with group work and the specific types of interaction were also important. It was also noted that the weak and average students benefited most from the group interaction, even when there were no "good" students in the group.

Lochhead and his colleagues (Lochhead, 1985; Whimbey & Lochhead, 1980, 1981) have used pair problem solving to increase the active involvement of students in learning and thus bring about a substantive change in how students view their own learning strategies. Throughout their school career, children are taught to listen or read and memorize. Rarely are they encouraged to generate ideas. Lochhead's program involves the interaction of pairs of students, each performing a different but complementary role. While one reads and thinks aloud, the other listens and constantly checks the steps of problem solution for accuracy. In this way, the students become very aware of and actively involved in the problem solving process. Putting their thoughts into words also reveals sloppy thinking and forces them to clarify their ideas. The teacher acts as a type of coach, monitoring the behavior of the pairs, giving feedback and prompting only when necessary. The teacher's role has been described as a type of Socratic dialogue, challenging and asking pertinent questions rather then offering solutions. The goal is for each student to be able to perform both roles at the same time (i.e., to listen to himself thinking and to think when listening to someone else). The problem of evaluating the outcomes of these programs is discussed at length by Lochhead (1985). This is clearly a difficult area because we are talking about radical, wide-ranging changes in learning behavior.

A similar series of experiments in cooperative learning strategies has investigated the effects of a number of aspects of group interaction (O'Donnell et al., 1985; Spurlin, Dansereau, Larson, & Brooks, 1984), based on a learning strategy program developed by the same group (Dansereau et al., 1979). Pairs of students were instructed to learn passages of text by alternating the roles of reader and summarizer. A significant feature of the method was the metacognitive activity (detecting errors and omissions) of the reader during his partner's summarization. This strategy proved superior to individual learning and to that of pairs who developed their own method. The summarization role was more effective than a passive listener role, but when the listener took a more active facilitating role, the performance of both partners was enhanced (Spurlin et al., 1984). Unfortunately, the actual elaborations were not recorded.

One of the interesting features of these studies and those of Lochhead is the facilitative role of metacognitive activity. Larson and co-workers (1985) attempted to separate the effects of metacognitive activity from those of elaboration, and found that while the former increased cooperative learning, transfer to individual learning was facilitated by the latter. It has been suggested that one of the functions of the group is to make overt many of the executive functions usually hidden when an individual works alone. This type of "other-regulation" is especially important for less mature or less capable learners. The role of critic and evaluator first learned in the interpersonal setting can then become internalized as a self-regulatory skill (Brown & French, 1979).

This discussion has covered quite a wide range of theory and experimentation, in search of the variables implicated in the relative effectiveness of group interaction. One of the problems encountered in such a survey is the number of dimensions involved in each study, and the resulting difficulty in making valid comparisons. Group problem-solving studies have used children of all ages and adults, ability levels ranging from retarded to gifted, various sizes of groups, combinations involving all sorts of homogeneous and heterogeneous groupings, and an endless variety of tasks.

We have already mentioned some studies involving low-ability children in which group discussion, in groups both with and without more able children, has been more effective than individual learning (Kol'tsova, 1978; Smith et al., 1981). Different findings have been shown in experiments in which various combinations of high-, medium-, and low-ability students work together on a concept mastery test in dyads or triads (Laughlin, Branch, & Johnson, 1969). The authors theorize that a person possesses all the resources of a person of lesser ability, but not necessarily the same resources as a person of comparable ability. Groups can only exceed the performance of individuals when pooling unshared resources. It follows from these presuppositions that low-achieving subjects should benefit from working in groups with any other individuals, but those of higher ability will only benefit from working with those at least as capable. Although some of these predictions were upheld in these experiments, less benefit was found from combining middle-ability than high-ability students, and low-ability students performed better alone than with other low-ability students. Johnson and co-workers (1981) pointed out that within cooperative groups, the more heterogeneous the participants and the more skilled they are at combining different items of information, the more likely the occurrence of constructive controversy. These conditions are less likely to be met within homogeneous low-ability groups, which may help explain the findings for low-ability students in the Laughlin studies.

Johnson and Johnson (1986) have discussed these issues from the perspective of the benefits to be gained from the inclusion of handicapped children in mainstream study groups. Although they have focused principally on attitudes and relationships, which are considerably enhanced by cross-handicap interaction, our main interest here is the effect of such groupings on the learning and cognitive growth of the handicapped students. In a meta-analysis of all relevant research studies from 1924 to 1981, Johnson and co-workers (1981) found that students of all ability levels demonstrated higher achievements and greater retention of learning as a result of participation in cooperative learning groups. They also tended to use higher-level thought processes, more high-level oral rehearsal, and higher-level learning strategies.

Obviously, it is not enough just to talk about the effectiveness (or otherwise) of group interaction; it is essential to look closely at the actual interactions involved. The processes by which the cognitive effects of group interaction are mediated are not always clear, but only by examining those processes can we begin to understand the parameters of group effects. A number of experiments on group or team learning have been carried out to examine more closely the interaction occurring in groups. We will offer a brief survey of these findings; for more extensive reviews, the reader is referred to Johnson and co-workers (1981), Sharan (1980), and Webb (1982).

Passive listening to other children's solutions does not improve performance (Webb, 1980), and vocalizing to demonstrate mastery of material is not as effective as vocalizing to teach other students (Durling & Schick, 1976). Bargh and Schul (1980) suggest that preparing to teach someone else necessitates producing a more organized cognitive structure than learning for oneself (as we saw in the previous discussion on peer tutoring). From the recipient's point of view, receiving explanations in response to questions relates positively to achievement, whereas receiving restated solutions without explanation has a negative effect (Webb, 1982). Receiving help from high-ability children is only effective when the assistance is in response to a stated need; on the other hand, children in homogeneous low-ability groups may fail to get their questions answered at all, a situation strongly predictive of failure (Webb, 1982). For these reasons, heterogeneous groups emphasizing helping behavior, especially the giving and receiving of high-order explanations, may be most beneficial to low- and high-ability rather than medium-ability children (Peterson, Janicki, & Swing, 1981; Swing & Peterson, 1982).

The question of transfer from the group to the individual situation is also relevant here, since improved performance by the group does not necessarily increase subsequent performance by the individual child (Hudgins, 1960). Transfer of group learning effects is also dependent on the efforts of the most able child to communicate his or her knowledge. In addition, outcome variables such as achievement measures and social/affective measures may be differentially affected by cooperative learning (Martino & Johnson, 1979).

Social Skills of Learning-Disabled Children

Much of the research into group processes has focused on group problem solving. Group interaction is also of interest in its own right, especially in terms of effective communication. Recent interest in the social skills and low social status of learning-disabled children has included investigation of deficits in behavior, social perceptiveness, nonverbal communication, and language skills (Dudley-Marling & Edmiaston, 1985). Much attention has been focused on the pragmatic skills of learning-disabled children, that is, their use of language in social situations. A seemingly large body of evidence has accumulated implicating pragmatic deficits in the poor social performance of learning-disabled children (Bryan & Bryan, 1978; Donahue, Bryan, & Pearl, 1980; Soensken, Flagg, & Schmits, 1981). For example, Donahue and colleagues (1980) found learning-disabled children more likely to agree and less likely to disagree with other members of their group, and less likely to monitor the group's progress. However, a number of studies have failed to replicate these findings (Markoski, 1983; Olsen, Wong, & Marx, 1983). Boucher (1984) found that despite a slight lag in verbal language complexity in learning-disabled children, they were as likely as non-learning-disabled children to adapt their language to the age of a listener. They also made more statements that encouraged cooperation, showed a greater tendency to promote joint problem solving, and made more questioning statements. A review by Dudley-Marling (1985) pointed out serious weaknesses in many of the original experiments in terms of sample selection, sample size, and statistical procedures, which cast doubt on findings of pragmatic skill deficits in disabled learners.

In one particular area, effective communication, findings of deficits in learning-disabled children have been consistent and persuasive. Studies using a referential communication paradigm, in which children describe items from a set to enable listeners to select the matching item, showed less accurate communications on the part of learning-disabled subjects (Noel, 1980; Spekman, 1981). Learning-disabled children were also less effective in teaching a six-step operation to open a box (Feagans, 1980) and in responding to requests for clarification when teaching checkers to an adult (Knight-Arest, 1984).

6
How Can I Know What I Think Till I See What I Say?

We began this survey of the spontaneous strategic behavior of handicapped children with a discussion of some of the differences in cognitive processes between handicapped and nonhandicapped learners. Competent learners produce a variety of strategies, depending on task demands, whereas ineffective learners tend not to generate their own strategies in the absence of adult guidance. Transfer or generalization has been noted many times to be particularly difficult for handicapped students; when the student is presented with a new and slightly different task, the previous knowledge is either not applied or is applied exactly as taught, without adaptation to the requirements of the new situation.

The research literature has supported the characterization of handicapped learners as unable to transfer or generalize information from one situation to another (Brown, 1978). Attempts to improve memorization have generally focused on training a single strategy such as rehearsal (Butterfield, Wambold, & Belmont, 1973), verbal mediation (Jensen & Rohwer, 1963), or elaboration (Campione & Brown, 1974). Although these interventions have met with some success in improving recall immediately after training, little has been achieved in terms of transfer (Burger, Blackman, & Clark, 1981; Campione & Brown, 1974). One of the reasons proposed to explain this consistent finding is that different kinds of problems or stimuli require at least slightly different applications of a given strategy.

We have discussed at some length our belief that one of the main difficulties in achieving transfer of learning by handicapped children is our failure as teachers to take sufficient account of children's preferred and spontaneous learning styles and the varying strategic requirements of different tasks. The procedure of training a handicapped learner in the use of a "good" strategy might result in a rigid expectation that it is the sole appropriate solution regardless of task demands. By contrast, adequate problem solvers are flexible in their approach to learning and can modify previously learned strategies in response to novel stimulus demands (Battig, 1975). Although disabled learners can be trained to produce their own elaborative responses in a specific learning situation (Pressley, 1982), little is known about their capacity to produce and select from a variety of possible strategies, some of which may be more appropriate to certain tasks and situations than others. A recent investigation (described at some length in Chapter 3) provided some evidence that learning-disabled children do benefit from a dual-strategy training intervention (Cherkes-Julkowski et al., 1986).

This chapter will describe some of our experimental efforts to look at the unprompted strategic behavior of different types of children on a simple memory task. Some of the preliminary findings obtained from a pilot study have already been discussed in Chapter 3. In essence, we were impressed by the evidence that handicapped children frequently approached the task in a very different fashion from that of average or gifted learners, and that their seemingly inefficient processing was not necessarily counterproductive for them. We agree with Bruner's conclusion, ". . . If one of our objectives is indeed to help people be good at problem solving, we had better keep well in mind how people would *like* to go at it, if they could get away with it" (1985, p. 599).

To overcome the difficulty of measuring strategy use (discussed in Chapter 4), we used small groups and recorded their discussions. We became concerned, however, that the encouragement of verbalization and active participation in the group dynamics might in itself have an effect on the strategic behavior of the children (Forman & Cazden, 1985; Skon, Johnson, & Johnson, 1981). We therefore included a sample of children examined individually, using the "talk aloud" method, so that we could compare the behavior of children working alone with that of children in groups.

The sample for this study consisted of 137 students from several comparable nonurban school districts in Connecticut. Children in four diagnostic categories, average, learning disabled, slow learning, and gifted, with a mean mental age between 8.0 and 9.0 years were included. For the purpose of this experiment, these categories were operationally defined as follows.

Average: Children performing in the fourth to sixth stanine or with IQ scores in the range of 85 to 115 on school-administered standardized tests and not in any special or remedial program.
Learning Disabled: Children identified by the school system as learning disabled and having an IQ in the range of 85 to 115.
Slow Learning: Children performing in the first to third stanines on school-administered standardized tests or with IQs in the range of 55 to 80. Most of these children were included in special programs for the educationally handicapped.
Gifted: Children performing in the eighth to ninth stanines on school-administered standardized tests having IQ scores above 125 or identified by the school system as gifted. (Gifted learning-disabled children were not included in this sample.)

Children in each diagnostic category were randomly assigned to one of two conditions, group or individual, with the restriction that chronological ages in the two conditions were as close as possible. Children within a school district were assigned across the two treatment conditions.

Children were presented with a memory problem in which they were asked to memorize pairs of pictures, each pair presented on a single card with one picture above the other. Three sets of pictures were used, each consisting of paired stimuli designed to appeal to a different strategy for memorizing and recalling the second member of the pair. The three types of stimuli were as follows.

Similarities: Pairs of common objects that could be combined under a single classification label (e.g., flower, different flower; dog, different dog).

Sentential: Two common objects from different categories that could be linked
with a sentence. Pairs of objects were chosen for which such a connection could
be made fairly easily, but not automatically (e.g., girl and apple).

Abstract: Pairs of abstract, nonrepresentational forms that could be labeled by
using the subject's interpretation (e.g., abstract shape resembling an oval and
abstract shape resembling a cube).

Single cards depicting the top picture from each pair and a large card displaying
all the bottom pictures arranged in random order (posttest array) were used for
posttesting. The posttest array and an example pair from each stimulus type are
shown in Figure 6.1.[1] In addition, a separate sample array together with one
sample pair card and the equivalent single card were used to demonstrate the task
and ensure comprehension. A complete set of stimulus pictures is included in
Appendix A.

Different procedures were followed for the two treatment conditions, group
and individual. Directions were developed and revised to be equivalent for the
two conditions, to promote understanding of the task, and, in the group condition, to stimulate discussion.

Group Condition

Children were examined in homogeneous groups of three children from the same
diagnostic category. Directions were as follows.

We're going to play a team game. Do you know what teamwork is? (Wait, try to elicit a
response from each child.) Right, teamwork is when you work together. In our game you're
going to work together as a team to remember some pairs of pictures. Who knows what
pair means? (Wait, try to elicit the idea of "goes together.") Right, a pair is two things that
go together. Look at this pair. (Present sample pair card.) Your job is to remember that this
one (point to bottom) goes with this one (point to top). Later, I'll show you just this one
(top) and you'll need to show me which picture goes with it. Let's try it. Look at these.
Now (display sample response array and top stimulus picture), which picture goes with
this one? Good. Now, who can tell me what you're supposed to do? (Ascertain that each
child understands the task.)

OK. Now is the time for the teamwork. Here are some pairs of pictures. The three of you
need to work together and decide the *best* way to remember these pairs. Take your time
and discuss it. We will listen, but we won't give any hints. When you've finished we'll see
if you can remember which pairs of pictures went together. Any questions? OK, let's get
started.

The examiner presented the pairs one at a time. Within each diagnostic category, the order of presentation of the stimulus types was counterbalanced to

---

[1]Drawings were done by Johanna Sayre.

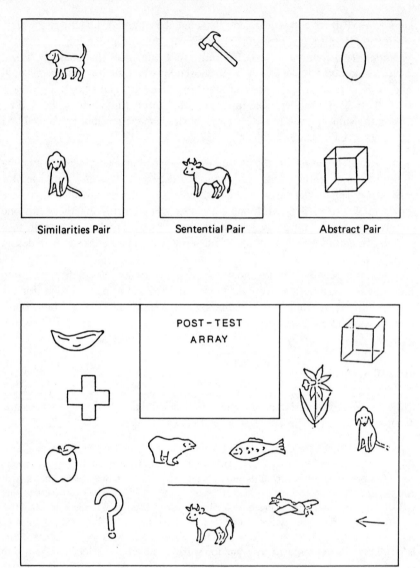

Similarities Pair   Sentential Pair   Abstract Pair

FIGURE 6.1.

reduce positional effects and the likelihood of a "strategy set" being established. Probing (i.e., using such comments as, "What is the best way to remember that these two go together?") was used only when no response was forthcoming. The children were allowed to discuss each card until they signaled that they had finished.

One of the authors and two other experimenters, trained to make verbatim transcriptions, were present at each session, each person responsible for recording the complete verbalizations of one child and abbreviated comments of the other children. This method had been found the most satisfactory for obtaining a complete record of the session, since it proved impossible for one person to record all utterances. Tape recording was found to be unsatisfactory because the tendency for children in groups to speak simultaneously produced undecipherable tapes.

Individual Condition

Each child was examined by the same experimenter. Directions were as follows.

We're going to play a game with some pairs of pictures. Do you know what *pair* means? (Wait, try to elicit the idea of "goes together.") Right, a pair is two things that go together. Look at this pair. (Display sample pair card.) Your job is to remember that this one (point to bottom) goes with this one (point to top). Later, I'll show you just this one (top) and you'll need to show me which picture goes with it. Let's try it. Look at these. Now (display sample response array and top stimulus picture), which picture goes with this one? Good. Now, can you tell me what you are supposed to do?

Now (indicate 12 pairs), here are some pairs of pictures. You need to decide the *best* way to remember these pairs. Take your time and tell me how you are going to do it. I'll listen, but I won't give any hints. When you've finished, we'll see if you can remember which pictures went together. Any questions? OK, let's get started.

The subject was encouraged to study each card, then signal readiness for the next. The experimenter wrote down everything said (including probes) and made note of any relevant behavior. Tape recording was not appropriate since it could not be used in the group condition and would have introduced an uncontrolled variation in procedure.

Posttest

Each subject was tested individually; in the group condition each of the three examiners tested one child, so that this could be done immediately after the discussion period. Subjects were shown each of the original 12 stimulus pictures in random order and asked to point to its associate on the response array. Success or failure was noted for each pair. The total score for each child out of a possible 12 correct responses was computed (posttest score).

A scoring system was developed to include every response obtained in the study. This resulted in 44 categories of responses (strategies). Categories were chosen to account for all of the responses with the minimum of scoring categories. Interrater reliability, as measured by percentage agreement between two experimenters on a sample of responses selected randomly from each diagnostic category and experimental condition, was 83%. Details of some of the most frequently used scoring categories, with abbreviations and examples, are given in Appendix B.

The three protocols for children within each group were combined to produce one script. All scripts were scored according to the above system, giving frequencies for each of the 44 strategies included in the scoring system.

Results and Discussion

The distribution of total scores by diagnostic category and experimental condition is shown in Table 6.1. The gifted children scored highest and the slow learners lowest, with the other two groups taking intermediate positions. Differences among all of the diagnostic categories were significant except that between the average and learning-disabled groups. Despite the findings of many studies that learning-disabled students have difficulty with memory tasks (Bauer, 1977), the learning-disabled children performed at a level equal to that of average learners in this particular type of associative memory task. This replicates previous findings using a similar procedure (Cherkes-Julkowski, Gertner, & Norlander, 1986).

The slow-learning group performed significantly more poorly than the other categories. They showed a wide range of performance, some obtaining the lowest scores of the sample (3 of 12), others showing perfect recall. The variability did not appear to relate directly to chronological age, which did not correlate with posttest score for any diagnostic category or to measured IQ, since some of the highest scores were obtained by children with the lowest IQs. Since IQ scores were not available for all children, it was not possible to correlate score and IQ. The significant factor in posttest performance appeared to be the type and combinations of mnemonic strategies produced by the children.

Considering the different types of stimuli separately, all diagnostic categories obtained high scores on the similarity pairs, the slow-learning group performed much more poorly on the other eight pairs, the gifted group maintained a fairly high level throughout, and the average and learning-disabled groups were intermediate. The difference between scores on the abstract and sentential stimuli was not significant for any diagnostic category.

For all diagnostic categories, similarities stimuli proved easier to recall than the other two stimulus types. This differential was especially marked in the slow-learning children. Jacoby, Bartz, and Evans (1978) have discussed the relationship between subject variables such as levels of processing and the potential meaningfulness of the material, both of which appeared to produce similar effects in terms of derived meaning. The relative ease of recall of the similarities pairs may be interpreted in terms of greater intrinsic "meaningfulness," even in the

TABLE 6.1. Distribution of mean posttest scores by category and condition [group (G) or individual (I)][a]

	Average		Gifted		Slow learners		Learning disabled	
	G	I	G	I	G	I	G	I
$M \pm SD$	10.9±1.1	9.1±1.9	11.1±1.0	11.3±1.9	6.3±2.2	7.2±2.3	10.1±1.7	10.3±1.7
Total ± SD	10.2±1.7		11.2±1.4		6.7±2.2		10.2±1.6	

[a] Maximum score = 12.

absence of deep levels of processing. Many of the average, gifted, and learning-disabled children commented that the similarities cards were easy, and some of the individuals restricted their discussion to one strategy (relevant similarities, "They both fly," or labeling similarities, "They're both airplanes"). It should be noted that although such similarity *strategies* were most frequently used for the similarity *stimuli*, they were also used for the sentential and abstract stimuli. For example, "They could both be on a farm" was used for the hammer/cow pair, and "They're both in the sky at night" for moon/cross (interpreted as star).

Average children were characterized by the high number of similarity strategies, both relevant (e.g., "They both swim") and irrelevant (e.g., "They're both small"), and by frequent use of developed differences (e.g., "You can eat a banana, but you can't eat a chair"). Gifted children also used similarities, but were exceptional in their awareness of visual similarities and differences and in noting subtle differences between otherwise similar stimuli, such as differences in leaf shape on the two flowers. They brought to the task a fund of general information (including references to Napoleon's hat, an eclipse of the moon, William Tell, the Big Apple, and many others) that facilitated the development of mnemonic strategies by allowing the integration of new and existing knowledge (Bransford et al., 1979). These children also demonstrated more metacognitive awareness (including understanding of the strategic requirements of the task) than all but the learning-disabled children. Remarks such as "Some of these are easy. . .the ones that are the same: dog–dog, fish–fish," or "The ones that are two things like each other are simple, but the others are kind of hard" were quite commonly made by gifted children.

Gifted children also showed the highest level of relevant connections, strategies that provided a specific association between the two stimulus pictures. These types of responses were many and varied, and some showed extraordinary creativity. There was a core of connections, however, that seemed to stem naturally from the stimuli and occurred over and over again: "The *girl* can eat the *apple*," "You could sit in the chair and eat the banana," "That's a *hook* and it can hang on the Christmas *tree*," and so forth.

By far the most intragroup agreement was shown by gifted groups (with the slow learners showing very little of this), and gifted children were responsible for almost all efforts to obtain agreement on a particular "best" strategy. The other groups were more inclined to consider whether they had finished or "discussed it enough." The following is a not untypical exchange from a group of slow learners:

J. I'm done, are you, S? Just look at it and see if you see anything else. You're not done with it yet?
S. Done?
J. He's not done yet? You just have to figure it out.
S. This can fit in here.
J. I didn't figure that out. You done? Oh, he's done.

The average and, to a lesser extent, the gifted groups showed very little off-task behavior, whereas the learning-disabled children were particularly noteworthy for their off-task behavior and irrelevant comments, which may account for their greater strategy production than any other category in both the group and individual conditions. However, they also showed a high level of metacognition and were more inclined to elaborate on responses than any other group. There were two basic differences between the types of metacognitions used by learning-disabled and gifted children. First, the gifted children showed more strategic awareness; their evaluative remarks were more concerned with finding ways to remember each pair, whereas the learning-disabled children talked extensively about the relative ease or difficulty levels. The second difference was that gifted children used many more control strategies in the group condition than when working individually. These strategies were frequently seen as efforts to plan a concerted approach:

> We're trying to figure out what . . . what do you think?
> How are we gonna remember this?

or as evaluative comments:

> That's a good one.
> No, everything here is shapes, so that won't do.

In contrast, learning-disabled children used more metacognitions in the individual condition. Many of the learning-disabled groups were so off task that they seemed unable to monitor their discussion at all.

Use of relevant connections was almost as frequent in learning-disabled as in gifted children and was highly correlated with successful performance. The quality of relevant connections used by the learning-disabled children was probably more variable than that of the gifted children, perhaps because a much wider range of ability was included in the former category. Although all the learning-disabled children scored within the average range on standardized tests, some of them appeared to be much brighter; their test scores may have been depressed by their learning difficulties. Apart from the more obvious associations such as "The *girl* can eat the *apple*," some of the children produced some very original ideas, which, on informal inspection, occur more often in the protocols of the gifted children. Some examples will give a sense of the possibilities:

The moon's hurt and it goes to the Red Cross hospital.
You could have a clock, and this would be one of the hands.
That could be a Frisbee and you're wrapping a present so the Frisbee could be in the box.
A dumb cow. Because if somebody had a hammer and hit the cow, it'd probably be dumb.
It's like a church my Dad designed. Inside like a cross, outside like the moon.
Let's see what we can do with the plus. Half moon plus half moon equals full moon.

The slow-learning children showed a tendency toward superficial processing (cf. Glidden et al., 1983) and a diminished knowledge base. Slow learners tended to use a lot of undeveloped strategies, including labeling, global statements of association or difference, and description of individual pictures. They were less likely than the other groups to form connections between the two stimuli and showed very little metacognitive awarenss. This was not true of all slow-learning children, however, and those who were able to develop associations between the stimuli were much more likely to show successful recall. The relevant connections produced by these children were less original than some of those developed by the more able students, but were equally effective. Slow learners also tended to be preoccupied with procedural concerns, such as whose turn it was next. This may well be because of the lack of familiarity of handicapped children with the group learning situation.

A factor analysis of the data extracted 16 factors, accounting for 72% of the variance. These factors showed a tendency for certain strategies to be used in concert, and the pattern of factor use among the diagnostic categories varied markedly. For example, one factor appears to include high-level strategies: relevant connections, elaborations, metaoperations, and agreement and disagreement. Gifted children scored highest on this factor, then the learning-disabled, avarage, and slow-learning groups in that order. Another factor deals with procedural concerns (instructions and turn-taking), on which slow learners scored highest. The slow-learning group also scored highest on the factor involving global associations and information questions. Irrelevant similarities, relevant similarities, and labeling similarities comprise a factor on which average children scored higher than the other three categories. Visual connections appear in a factor along with task-related and off-task irrelevancies; learning-disabled children obtained very high scores on these strategies. This factor analysis clarifies some of the patterns that distinguish among the diagnostic groupings.

Group and Individual Conditions

The strategies that most clearly discriminated between the individual and group conditions included some of those intrinsically related to group functioning (e.g., agree, disagree). Since children in the group condition used more than three times as many strategies as children in the individual condition, the remaining strategies were examined to find which departed from the expected frequency based on total strategy usage. Children in groups tended to focus on one stimulus, whereas individual children described both stimuli or attempted to find connections between them. Individual children were also more likely to ask labeling questions or to say they didn't know, to form undeveloped associations and differences, and to look for similarities rather than differences. The most likely explanation for this was that the pattern of responses in the groups tended to be first to describe the stimuli or find similarities or connections, and then go on to develop differences. The individual children did not usually go beyond the first stage. The role of group discussion in these cases was to prolong the strategy production, which was not necessarily either efficient or effective. Children in groups also showed more off-task discussion and more preoccupation with procedural concerns. The effect of these behaviors on posttest performance will be discussed further in the next section.

Relationship Between Strategy Usage and Performance

Results were also analyzed (using multiple regression techniques) to investigate which strategies predicted successful performance. Relevant connections and developed differences were most highly predictive of success in both individual and group conditions, whereas labeling similarities (e.g., "They're both flowers") predicted success in the individual condition only. Turn-taking and undeveloped differences predicted failure in the group condition, labeling one picture in the individual condition.

Different patterns of strategy use predicted performance for different diagnostic categories. For the average, slow-learning, and learning-disabled children, relevant connections were positively related to posttest score. Functional similarities (e.g., "You could use a cow and a hammer on a farm") served a positive role for average and learning-disabled children, whereas similarities and differences (e.g., "They're both dogs, but one's sitting and one's standing") were helpful to the average and slow-learning groups.

In general, then, the children who exhibited strategies directed at forming specific connections between pairs of stimuli (associative, differentiating, or elaborative) tended to show better recall. However, this relationship was not simple, since the strategies that predicted score varied widely among diagnostic categories. For average, gifted, and learning-disabled children, establishing a relevant connection between the two stimuli was the strategy that related most strongly and positively to successful performance. Although relevant connections were also predictive of success for the slow-learning group, the strategy that related most strongly to success for slow-learning children was word play, which established a striking and unique relationship between the *names* of the two pictures. The most frequent example of this was the *bear–cup* combination, for which discovery of the word play *cub–cup* invariably prompted recall. One slow learner also found the word play

> This is a hammer and this is made from ham. You get cow meat from ham.

There was an element of humor in these plays on words that was a striking mnemonic for all the children; it gave a real jolt to the slow learners, and unfortunately is probably not utilized in most of their learning environments. Other attempts at word play were less successful; for one gifted child, these efforts were so obscure as to be counterproductive:

> Trying to think of something on the bear that would rhyme with cup. You should handle a cup with care and this is a bear.

and

> You hammer nails and a cow has a tail. Nails and tails.

The effect of specific variables such as labeling or using visual cues appeared to depend on two distinct factors: how effective these were in identifying individual pictures and the extent to which they created a unique relationship between the two members of a pair (Stein, 1977). Verbal labeling has been shown to facilitate both recall (Hagen & Kingsley, 1968) and recognition (Nelson & Kosslyn, 1976) of previously presented pictures. Although labeling per se was frequently used by all categories, the slow-learning group was almost twice as liable as the other three categories to label both pictures without any further development, and this tended to be predictive of failure. Labeling stimuli as part of a more complex strategy facilitated recall; without the second, connecting step, labeling was ineffective. In the slow-learning children, labeling appeared to be inefficient, using up processing capacity necessary for developing associative strategies. The result was that the children became stuck at the labeling stage and were unable to move on to deeper levels of processing. For the other diagnostic categories, the labeling stage was more often a prelude to further strategy development or was omitted altogether, the labeling being incorporated into the association (e.g., "The *girl* can eat the *apple*"). On the other hand, omitting labeling altogether was not productive, since there was a positive relationship overall between labeling and recognition. Statements such as "she can eat it" were often not definitive enough to prompt recognition. Of the strategies that could be used with or without labels (e.g., "The cow can drink out of the cup" or "It can drink out of that"), slow learners labeled 44%, learning-disabled children 86%, average 88%, and gifted 94%. Within any category, the tendency to use labels tended to vary between one child and another; some children seemed almost deliberately to eschew the use of labels. Here are two series of such responses (not in order as presented), one from a gifted and one from a learning-disabled child:

Gifted child

Girl/apple:	"Both have skin."
Hammer/cow:	"They each can make noise."
Chair/banana:	"Each weigh—can be put on a scale."
Oval/box:	"Both a type of shape."
Moon/cross:	"Both shapes—all I can think of."

Learning-disabled

Moon/cross:	"One's on the night time and the other one's like when you do an 8 plus 9."
Hammer/cow:	"An animal and something to use."
Girl/apple:	"One's a person and one's a fruit to eat."
Cup/bear:	"One's something to drink out of and the other's kind of like an animal."
Chair/banana:	"One's something to sit on—the other's something healthy to eat."

Although the overall use of labels by learning-disabled children was equal to that of average children, it might be interesting to examine more closely whether children with some types of learning disabilities (e.g., language-related) would be more likely to be nonlabelers. For this we would need more diagnostic information than was available for this study.

Our findings regarding the inhibiting effect of simply labeling stimuli without further development are enlightening if we consider again the desirability of imposing our own interpretation of "good" strategy on the children. In our original study of dual-strategy training (Cherkes-Julkowski et al., 1986), described in Chapter 3, we trained the children to label the diagrams and repeat the names over on the so-called rehearsal pairs. Apparently, this was not a good strategy to encourage, and many children selected a better one when left to their own devices.

Attempts to use the visual aspects of stimuli proved generally unhelpful. The reason for this appeared to lie in the frequent failure of these strategies to produce a unique connection or differentiation between stimuli. Comments such as, "This one can fit in this one," or, "They both have a bit sticking out at the side," could apply to almost any picture. However, there were some occasions when specific visual connections proved very helpful. For example, the only successful recall of a nonsimilarities pair for one slow-learning child was prompted by the statement "The hammer looks like the cow's tail." Apparently, for this child, using a visual association could produce a relevant and discriminating connection. It should be pointed out, however, that this association was formulated verbally; perception of this relationship may not have produced the same effect in the absence of an explicit verbal control strategy. As with labels, visualization was seen repeatedly in the protocols of specific children; in fact, some of the children most prone to using visual strategies were also nonlabelers:

Moon/cross: "The points are like those points on the end."
Hammer/cow: "Thing on the end looks like his horns."
Fish/fish: "This one has a longer fin than that one."
Dog/dog: "Both look sad."

Again, without more diagnostic information, we can only make guesses about the significance of these findings. However, it seems possible that "visual" children, perhaps those with weaker language skills, are more inclined to use "visual" strategies and that these may be more effective for them than for children with stronger verbal abilities. It would certainly be interesting to examine this relationship.

Agreement with another child predicted success for average children but failure for gifted and slow-learning children. In the slow-learning groups, agreement may have indicated lack of active involvement in the task, with the result that they were sometimes too quick to accept other children's ideas without sufficient attention to the material. There is no obvious reason why agreement should have been counterproductive for the gifted groups.

Labeling questions related positively to performance for the gifted and slow-learning but negatively for the learning-disabled children. In the gifted groups, labeling questions were quite common and were always responded to appropriately. Labeling questions were less frequently asked in the handicapped groups. Overall, however, labeling questions were much more often asked by children tested individually. The gifted children often answered their own questions:

This is an egg—or what? Is it anything I want? Then it's a cookie and it goes in the box.
Is this a banana? Well, it's gonna be.
Don't know what this is called. It's a question mark because I don't know what it is.
Is that a ball? If that was a soccer ball, some soccer balls come in boxes from the store.

It is hard to see why labeling questions might have predicted success for the slow learners, since we have already seen that simple labeling did not. It is possible that this finding is spurious, since labeling questions tended to be asked by the more successful slow learners. The finding that asking labeling questions was counterproductive for the learning-disabled children is also hard to account for; it may have occurred because the questions focused attention on the labeling process rather than on forming associations:

> Is this a bear? A bear and a cup.
> Is that a zigzag? I just would think of question, zigzag.

Metacognition

It was expected that metacognitive comments would be more common among higher-ability groups, and that this awareness of the superordinate aspects of the task would be related to successful performance. This prediction was only partially borne out. Gifted and learning-disabled children were much more likely to show metacognitive awareness than the other two categories. This finding is unexpected in view of the suggestion that learning-disabled children perform poorly on deliberate memory tasks because they do not plan effectively (Torgesen & Licht, 1983). However, Sternberg and Wagner (1982) have proposed that learning disabled children remain at the stage of consciously directed behavior longer than average learners. This seemed to apply to the disabled learners in this sample; their metacognitive comments tended to be much less planful and more concerned with ongoing activity.

One gifted child was unusual in his awareness of the need to tailor his memorization to the requirements of the posttest, with several comments such as:

They're both dogs—if she's gonna show the big card and lots of pictures. If she has a couple of dogs, then you have to remember sitting and standing.

Similarly, the following interaction took place in a gifted group:

J. Can you stop writing, please. I can't remember all these.
M. You might be able to when you see the board.
J. Can I see the board, please?

For some groups, metacognitive remarks tended to increase when the children were having difficulty finding a satisfactory strategy or when they developed a "response set," producing the same type of strategy over and over again, which occurred frequently in all but the gifted groups. For example, one learning-disabled group could not break out of a pattern of expressing differences:

C. Don't just give differences. You're saying what the difference is. She wants to know what's alike in them.
E. All along I've been telling 'em differences?
P. A bear has ears and a cup doesn't.
E. Stop telling 'em differences.

C. I can't, they're not even anything living.
P. The bear has bumps, the cup doesn't.
C. You're telling the differences; she asked for what's the same.
P. That's dumb. I can't think of anything else.

Examples of strategy set were quite rare, however, even in the handicapped groups.

Group Interaction

Group interaction stimulated a great deal of verbalization, which resulted in long sessions, but was not necessarily productive. Time alone may not lead to effective learning:

Time may be a correlate of memory to the extent that time is necessary for processing to some level, but it is possible that further time spent in merely recycling the information after this optimal level will not predict trace durability (Craik & Lockhart, 1972, p. 681).

Much of the verbalization in groups appeared to be this type of repetitive recycling, without development of deeper levels of processing, especially in the slow-learning groups. These children appeared so unused to the experience of working in a small group that they had great difficulty focusing on the task at all. Only one slow-learning child in the group condition produced relevant connections, whereas 7 of 14 in the individual condition did so. The production of a relevant connection seemed to be facilitative whether it was the only response or was embedded in less productive discussion.

Group interaction played a positive role for average children, as evidenced by the superior performance of children in the group condition and by the positive association between interactive comments and successful performance. One possible reason for this may have been the greater use of both relevant connections and word play by average children in the group condition, whereas all other diagnostic categories used both of these strategies more in the individual condition. For the gifted children, for whom the task was relatively easy, individual mnemonic behavior was effective without the additional processing produced by group interaction. Learning-disabled children performed equally well in the group and individual conditions. They used more relevant connections in groups than any other category. No evidence was seen of difficulties in pragmatic skills (cf. Dudley-Marling, 1985); their patterns of agreement, disagreement, group processing and questioning were very similar to those of the average and gifted children. As mentioned previously, the monitoring of group problem solving by learning-disabled children, as measured by metacognitive comments, was second only to that of the gifted groups. The passive style of learning attributed to learning-disabled children (Torgesen, 1982) was not seen in this study. Boucher (1984) has suggested that learning-disabled children take a passive role only when the appropriate response strategy is unclear to them, perhaps in academic or other symbolic tasks. We considered the possibility that active involvement in the task (at least in terms of metacognitive comments) was the result of an energizing effect of participating in a group; this is unlikely, since this behavior was seen more frequently in the learning-disabled children tested individually.

Responses to Different Stimulus Types

We have referred several times to our belief in the importance of recognizing and adjusting to differences in task demands, in order to select the most appropriate strategies, rather than applying the same strategies in a rigid and suboptimal fashion. We were particularly interested in the ability of handicapped children to differentiate among the three stimulus types and in the way in which their choices of "best" strategy related to success or failure in memorization.

For each diagnostic category, discrimination between the stimulus types on the basis of strategy usage was extremely high (discriminant function tests). Differentiation in both handicapped groups was a little less clear than in the average and gifted groups.

Some interesting patterns emerged regarding the differential use of strategies by the four categories of subjects on the three types of stimulus cards. Strategies that discriminated between stimulus types were not necessarily those most frequently used. For example, developed differences was one of the most commonly used strategies overall, but did not prove highly discriminating, since it was used for all stimulus types.

The strategy that most clearly differentiated between stimulus pairs was relevant connections, which was used most frequently for the sentential cards. For the slow-learning group, functional description of both pictures was also highly discriminating and was used mainly for the similarities stimuli. Visual connection was another strategy that was highly discriminating, especially for the average and gifted groups. This strategy was used most often on the abstract cards (e.g., "The oval can fit in the box") and was used more frequently by the learning-disabled group than the other diagnostic categories. This finding is particularly interesting in view of attempts to identify subcategories of learning-disabled children, including those with language difficulties and those with visual perceptual problems (Boder, 1971; Denckla, 1972). Unfortunately, we do not have diagnostic information about our learning-disabled sample and are unable, therefore, to examine the possible relationship between our findings of choice of visual connections as a mnemonic strategy and language-related disabilities.

Other strategies that discriminated between stimulus types were relevant similarities for the average and slow-learning groups and visual similarities for the average, gifted, and slow-learning groups, although this strategy was used much more frequently by the gifted children than by those in any other diagnostic category. Relevant similarity was most frequently used for the similarities pairs and visual similarity for the sentential pairs (e.g., "The hammer looks like the cow's tail"). Labeling similarity was used exclusively for the similarities pairs and was most strongly discriminating for the gifted group. Irrelevant similarity was highly discriminating for the average and gifted groups, who tended to use this strategy for the abstract stimuli (e.g., "They're both shapes").

On the whole, similarities pairs were easiest to remember, and this could be done by using a similarity strategy ("They're both dogs, flowers," and so forth). In the individual condition, gifted and slow-learning children used fewer strategies on the similarity cards, whereas in the group condition, only gifted children did so. Some children worked to stop unnecessary discussion by their groups on these pairs by advocating simplicity:

Gifted group
E. Both doing something, walking and sitting. Both dogs.
N. This one's walking.
C. No, this dog that's sitting down called this one to come and play.
E. That's too complicated.
C. It is?
E. Yeah. They're both dogs.
N. OK. They're both dogs. That's settled.

Prediction of performance on the similarities cards was inhibited by perfect or near-perfect scores for these stimuli by all but the slow-learning group. In the latter group, attempts to find differences between the pairs entered the regression equation; undeveloped differences and visual differences predicted failure, and developed differences predicted success.

The sentential and abstract stimuli required greater use of associative strategies to derive meaning from the stimulus pairs. Producing these strategies and consequently remembering the pairs was difficult for the slow learners but not for the learning-disabled children. On the abstract pairs, success was predicted by relevant connections for all categories but the slow-learning children.

Slow-learning children tended to do more labeling on the sentential and especially the abstract pairs, and also to be much more likely to focus on one member of the pair. Visual description of one picture was most frequently seen on the abstract pairs, functional description of one picture on the sentential stimuli. Undeveloped differences (e.g., "They're not the same") were also quite common on the abstract and sentential pairs, whereas developed differences were much more frequent on the similarity stimuli. Both relevant connections and word play were most frequently seen and were the best predictors of success on the sentential pairs, although the absolute number of these connections was very small compared to the other diagnostic categories. This pattern of strategic behavior seems to demonstrate the awareness of the slow-learning children that abstract and sentential pairs needed a different approach than similarities, and the beginning of an attempt to respond to this need.

Learning-disabled children showed a much wider range of strategies in dealing with the abstract and sentential stimuli and used extensive elaboration of ideas in an attempt to come up with "good" strategies. Relevant connections were predictive of success on both the abstract and sentential pairs, whereas the off-task behaviors involved in irrelevant comments and remarks such as, "I was going to say that" and "I already said that" were predictive of failure on the abstract pairs. Discrimination between stimuli was somewhat less clear-cut than in the average and gifted groups, which may be taken as an indication of some inflexibility or failure to examine task demands sufficiently, but overall score was at an identical level to that of average children.

Although the similarities stimuli produced the highest scores in all categories, some of the abstract and sentential pairs proved easier to develop associations for and easier to recall than others. The *girl–apple* combination ("The girl can eat the apple") was perfectly recalled by gifted children and produced highest scores among the nonsimilarities pairs overall. Of the abstract pairs, *oval–box* was easiest to recall by all but the slow-learning children, who were more successful with *tree–question mark*. A number of slow-learning children called the oval a circle, which may have caused confusion with the *circle–arrow* pair. *Circle–arrow* proved to be the most difficult pair to deal with for all categories, although there was no difficulty labeling either of the stimuli. In fact, this was the only abstract pair that was easily labeled by most children. It is possible that labels were chosen for the other abstract stimuli in conjunction with consideration of their pairings; for example, the oval was frequently called an egg because it fit in the box, the cross was called a star because of its association with the moon, and the question mark was called a hook to fit on the Christmas tree. Because of the ease of labeling the circle and arrow, the push to find a connection was less evident in this case, and many children did not go beyond the labeling stage, which may have resulted in difficulty of recall on the posttest. This is another indication that ease of labeling in itself is less important than making a connection between the labels.

When responses to different stimulus types were assessed separately, the effect of metaoperations was seen in the ability of task awareness (e.g., in assessing the relative difficulty of the three stimulus types) to predict success for the average and slow-learning groups on the abstract pairs and of strategic awareness (i.e., discussion of favored strategies) for average children on the abstract pairs and for gifted children on sentential pairs. Despite their high level of monitoring, metacognitive comments did not predict performance for learning-disabled children. This adds credence to the suggestion that these remarks performed more of a monitoring than a directing function.

It has been suggested (DeLoache, 1984) that more metacognitive behaviors are seen when a child is aware that the task is difficult. Since the abstract pairs proved most challenging for all diagnostic categories, awareness of this difficulty may have promoted greater effort on the part of some children, especially average and slow learners. The comment, "This one's hard" frequently accompanied success on abstract pairs. For the gifted children, sequences such as, "How do they both go together? A chair can get broken and a banana can get squashed," or "There are animals at the bottom of teacups–that'll help me remember," were common. The relationship between focus on the requirements of the task and production of a sentential relationship is also seen in the following exchanges from a gifted group:

C. How are we gonna remember this?
A. Bears don't drink from cups.
M. That's a good one.
C. Yeah, good one.

and

C. How are we gonna remember this?
A. The girl sat on a chair eating a banana.
M. We could do that.
A. Want to, C?
C. OK.

   By contrast was the average group, which tried to find similarities between all 12 pairs, rather than differentiate between strategies for different stimulus types.

L. What does a banana have in common with a chair? Only thing I can think of is you use them both.
A. You don't use a banana, you eat it.
L. That's like using it, isn't it?

However, there was sufficient flexibility of strategy selection overall to produce excellent discrimination between stimulus types for all diagnostic categories. The ability to apply different strategies in response to perceived differences in task demands, even though the children were not alerted to these differences in stimulus types, suggest that children from a wide range of ability levels spontaneously apply superordinate control processes, even when these are not made explicit. In general, apart from a few examples of "strategy set," even the slow-learning children tended not to transfer strategies rigidly from one stimulus pair to the next, but to deal with each new pair as a new situation requiring appropriate action. The problem for the slow-learning children was not in flexibility, but in being able to respond to the requirements of the more demanding situation by producing facilitative strategies.

Summary and Implications

One of the most striking findings of this study was the difference in mnemonic behavior among all four diagnostic categories. As we had hypothesized, when allowed to produce their own spontaneous cognitive strategies, handicapped children have their own way of doing things. However, it also appeared that many of the strategies that were most often used by the handicapped groups did not result in successful memorization. On the contrary, the more similar their behavior was to that of the gifted group, the better they did in the posttest. This generalization requires some modification, however, since some specific strategies were facilitative for the handicapped but not for the average or gifted children. Word play, for example, was strikingly effective for the slow learners, and visual similarities for the learning disabled. The combination of strategies could also be significant;

although a simple similarity strategy could be enough for a gifted child, the slow learner may benefit from the longer interaction with the stimulus implied in more complex and prolonged strategy production.

Results of this study validate the current approach to learning-disabled students as a distinct group, whose achievement in school subjects may be poor but whose performance in this paired-associate memory task was equivalent to that of average students, despite differences in strategic behavior. This is important in view of the current debate regarding the existence of learning disabilities as a valid concept (Sabatino, 1983).

The learning-disabled sample in this study showed a distinct pattern of strategic behavior, including a high level of elaboration and metacognitive awareness and an active involvement in the task that belied conceptualizations of learning-disabled students as passive learners (Torgesen, 1982). In fact, learning-disabled children behaved more like gifted or average than like slow-learning children, despite current emphasis on the slow-learner instructional model in programs for the learning-disabled. If such children are indeed passive in their approach to schoolwork, this may be a specific response to expectations of failure and feelings of inadequacy in tasks where they are at a disadvantage. Given a situation where they can succeed, learning-disabled children show a very different pattern of behavior. In addition, prescribed ways of approaching a task may encourage passivity. In many special education programs, learning tasks are structured in such a way that children need only move through them in a prescribed manner to experience guaranteed success. The hidden agenda for these students is not to encourage them to be independent learners, but to be successful producers. They are discouraged from developing their own learning approaches and, as we have discussed at length, from learning from their mistakes. The results of this study imply that attempts should be made to create learning situations that give learning-disabled children a feeling of choice and control over a task and teaching strategies that create a sense of competence and active involvement in learning.

The learning-disabled sample in our study also showed the distractibility and off-task behavior that has been considered a characteristic of these children. This type of behavior tended to predict failure on this task, and underlined the importance of creating a structured environment designed to minimize distraction. In our pilot study, however, we also noted that elaborations that were quite far-flung and off the point could be facilitative for the learning-disabled children. Perhaps there is a relationship between what we saw then as playing around with ideas and the metacognition we recorded so frequently in the later study. Apparently there is a fine line between what is relevant in terms of developing ideas and what is irrelevant and distracting. This whole area seems to need some closer investigation, as it seems to touch on something of importance for the education of learning-disabled children.

The slow-learning children in this study differed in many ways from the other three diagnostic categories. Although they performed more poorly overall, their success on the similarities stimuli showed that, given meaningful material to learn, they were capable of performing well. These children recognized the need to produce different types of strategic behavior when attempting to memorize the abstract and sentential stimuli, and awareness of the difficulty of this task sometimes promoted the development of facilitative associations. On the sentential pairs in particular, many of the slow-learning children produced relevant connections, which were highly correlated with success. These findings all support the view that appropriate instruction will emphasize flexibility of strategy use rather than rote implementation of strategies that cannot easily be transferred to different tasks and situations. The fact that many similar strategies were as helpful to the slow-learning children as to those in the other categories suggested that they do not need a radically different type of teaching; it may be better to teach them to use high-level associative strategies that they do not necessarily produce regularly or spontaneously. We have also noted specific counterproductive strategies that were used far more frequently by slow learners than by those in the other categories, in particular global associations and differences ("They're the same" or "They're different") and strategies that focused on one picture. Working with these children might involve helping them attend to more specific similar and different features, and to both stimuli rather than just one.

As with our learning-disabled sample, we found a wide spread among the slow learners, both in their ability to use high-level strategies and in their recall, but we could not relate either of these findings to differences in intelligence or to obvious genetic factors such as Down's syndrome. One little girl with Down's syndrome produced a record full of original and appropriate associations, although her speech was so poor it was hard to understand what she was saying. She also showed quite good recall. If we are to draw any practically applicable conclusions from our findings, we need to examine much more closely what makes one clearly impaired child able to function so successfully on an open-ended task *without any guidance*, whereas many others are unable to cope effectively.

It was hoped that the inclusion of gifted children in the study would show whether these children approached the task in a qualitatively different way from average and handicapped children. The gifted children did, in fact, show significantly higher posttest performance, in spite of a probable ceiling effect. These children made many associations using their broad knowledge base and showed a high level of metacognitive awareness that was more refined than that of the other groups, including a conscious awareness of the need to prepare in a specific manner for the posttest. However, the strategies used by gifted children were similar to those used by the other children, the differences being emphasis and quality. This implies that average and handicapped children could be taught to make better selections among the strategic choices available to them. In particular, the need for more active awareness of task demands and of the importance of task-appropriate processing could be emphasized.

One major question posed by this study was the relative effectiveness of group and individual problem solving. The average children, who were probably most familiar with the group learning situation, showed significant benefits from working with other children. Unlike those in the other diagnostic categories, average children produced more high-level associative strategies in the group condition, which was highly predictive of successful performance on the post-test. For the other categories, the group situation seemed to be more distracting then facilitative. For gifted children, the task was so easy that many of them could remember the pairs with minimal processing. The extra processing produced by the groups was not of benefit. Had the task been more difficult, however, a differential effect similar to that seen in the average groups might have emerged.

Neither of the handicapped groups showed a significant difference in perform-ance between the individual and group conditions. The slow-learning children were so preoccupied with the group process itself that they were not able to focus on developing mnemonic strategies. The learning-disabled children, on the other hand, became highly distracted and spent a great deal of group time in social interchange and off-task discussion. It is worth noting that in spite of their prob-lems in dealing with the group process, handicapped children performed as well in these circumstances as they did individually. Performance in the individual condition was more efficient, however, since group discussion involved much more processing time.

The results of this study do not, therefore, support the view that group interac-tion is facilitative for handicapped children. Nevertheless, since benefits were seen for children who *were* able to work well in groups, it may be premature to assume that handicapped children cannot be taught to function more effectively in small groups and to improve their strategic behavior through interaction with other children. Possible benefits can only be evaluated by exposing handicapped children to the group learning situation so that they can become more familiar with the process, then determining whether there are advantages to be gained by developing group interaction skills in these children.

7
Back to the Classroom

Flexible Programming

Throughout this discussion of cognitive strategies used by successful and less successful students, we have tried to keep one foot firmly in the classroom. After all, that is where theories and findings are put to the test. In this final chapter we will attempt to pull together some of the strands that have developed along the way and suggest some of the implications of our discussion for the education of children, especially those with learning problems. How can we best meet the needs of handicapped children, working with their natural inclinations rather than against them, while at the same time guiding them into more productive ways of using their abilities? One of the major issues to consider is the question of mainstreaming; however, this is not a simple "yes" or "no" matter. Mainstreaming is not an invariant entity; it is a plastic concept that can be (and is) molded to suit the beliefs and needs of any situation. It can mean lunch in the cafeteria, or checking in with the special education teacher and disappearing for the rest of the day. It is a topic that rouses strong feelings and is often politicized, the needs of the system frequently taking priority over those of the children. Our interest here is to include in our review a consideration of how education as a whole, including mainstreaming as well as other programmatic options, can best address some of the special characteristics of handicapped children, such as their need for mediated learning experiences and their difficulties in making use of group interaction.

Social Cognition and Group Instruction

Mediated learning can only take place in some kind of social context. A major focus of our work has been to consider the value of peer group interaction in the learning of children with educational handicaps, children who are slow learners or are learning disabled. Our results as well as those of others (Bryan, 1986) indicate that learning-disabled children perform as well but not better in small groups, whereas nonhandicapped children seem to be facilitated by the small peer group process. Despite the failure of group experiences to enhance strategic behavior as a whole, learning-disabled youngsters working in groups use more of the strategy type most predictive of success: relevant connections. There is, then, the potential for a strong positive effect of small group interaction. What is needed is a plan for greater exposure of these children to focused group interaction before asking them to use the group experience for the specific goal of content acquisition or learning how to learn. This exposure period might be thought of as an effort to desensitize learning-disabled children to the purely interpersonal and procedural aspects of working in groups. Traditionally, individualized and one-to-one instruction has been valued in special education, particularly for children with learning disabilities. Some individual instruction is certainly necessary given the combination of idiosyncratic processing styles and educational gaps of each child. Nevertheless, one goal of special instruction must be the development of metacognitive awareness, executive control, and strategy selection. The potential of social context for eliciting these processes is as great and possibly greater than that of other procedures tried thus far. Some systematic effort to desensitize learning-disabled children to the distracting effects of group interaction would be more than justified by this goal. At least one program that has emulated Feuerstein's mediated learning approach with middle and high school age learning-disabled youngsters has managed to orchestrate relatively large group interactions in which children act as mediators, external control agents, and personal support systems for each other (Stan-Spence & Spence, Ben Bronz Academy, West Hartford, CT, personal communication).

A planned approach to group interaction of this kind requires longitudinal programming toward the goal of working with others to enhance metacognitive and strategic behavior. Parents and school personnel would need to be willing to invest months into a process that might yield few immediate gains in skill acquisition, but would promise a rich return later. Furthermore, such a program raises the mainstream-related question about the nature of one's peer group. If handicapped children were to be grouped for "social cognition training" in sets of similarly slow-learning or learning-disabled students, this would require less time in the mainstream and would also imply identification with one's similarly disabled peers and less with nonhandicapped others in the mainstream.

Mediated learning, however, need not and should not depend only on peer interaction as defined by small groups of similarly diagnosed and functioning children. Our study did not address the question of the optimal kind of grouping. The social modeling literature suggests that the presence of one slightly advanced and more competent child would provide the target child with the appropriate view into the next higher level of functioning without it being overwhelming or simply beyond grasp. Peer in this case might be defined more broadly as, perhaps, one nonhandicapped among two handicapped learners. The educational advantages for the nonhandicapped learner would include the practice of metacognitive and interpersonal procedures; the organization and meta-awareness of one's own thoughts for the purpose of teaching others; and the opportunity to develop prosocial attitudes toward persons with handicaps. It is left to further investigation whether groups would function best if children were of the same gender, if this effect changes with age, and what the optimal age for such an intervention might be. Although we have considered the possible effects of gender in our research, we have not yet designed a study that controls for it.

Social Cognition and Apprenticeship

Instruction, however, should not depend solely on other children. The teacher–student social cognition context is clearly critical to the success of children with educational handicaps. Dyadic, individualized instruction of this kind stands in contrast to individualized instruction of the kind that is either one to one in a didactic arrangement or consists of identifying appropriate objectives and asks the learner to work independently until each is achieved. The goal of dyadic instruction would be to provide in the teacher the external executive control functions and the knowledge store through the teacher that is absent or not fully developed in the learner. Special instruction has long appreciated the need for externally imposed organization. Many Individualized Education Plans (IEPs) call for support in the resource room to help with organizational strategies and study skills. It is common practice to help children with outlining procedures, setting up study schedules, keeping notebooks, and the like. The external control and scaffolding is evident. Less evident in traditional dyadic approaches have been efforts to cede control by the teacher to the learner as happens in an apprentice–master relationship (Kaye, 1982a, 1982b). The apprentice takes part in a complete process that incorporates metacontrol by the master, use of previously learned content of the master, orchestration of strategy selection and use, and performance monitoring, direct experience, and practice, as well as the production of a successfully finished, material outcome.

Instruction that would follow this model, then, would need to begin in natural context and maintain the integrity of the whole process. In the example of a child who cannot become sufficiently organized for note taking, report writing, or perhaps even solving a two- or three-step mathematics problem, the principles of apprenticeship would apply in the following ways. The master/teacher would need to work interactively and supportively with the student. Although this does not absolutely require a one-to-one relationship, it does require that the teacher be aware of each move that the apprentice makes and whether the apprentice is ready for additional responsibility (i.e., working within the zone of proximal development). It also requires a supportive interpersonal relationship that is not threatened by too many demands made on the teacher by other students or by competition among the apprentices. Instruction would need to be embedded in the context of an actual problem, perhaps one arising out of the apprentice's own social or academic context. Starting with a clearly stated problem places the focus squarely on the outcome and how one might achieve it. In addition, the outcome has real, material, and personal value. The process can then begin, largely enacted during initial stages by the teacher, who does not make grandiose statements about abstracted principles or explicit rules for operating, but instead demonstrates the process in situ. For example, if the goal is to solve a multistep math problem, the teacher might ask the student to begin to solve it independently. This process often consists of verbalizing computations rather than writing them down. The teacher's role might be to demonstrate to the student how the student's operations look and work as written computations. From this point forward, the teacher's role would be to utilize existing processes to develop more accurate, more efficient, or perhaps more traditional approaches to solution. One student, for example, lacked automaticity with number facts involving larger amounts and more advanced operations. To figure how much money there would be if each of three people had four dollars, she divided the units of four in half and counted by twos. It would be the teacher's role to utilize such personally derived algorithms, to demonstrate what they would look like as calculations, and to move from this point to repeated additions with larger numbers and eventually multiplication. Only then might the teacher move to a more standard approach to problem solving. From this point forward, it would be important to use the same or similar problems in order for the apprentice to practice, and through practice to begin to assume control for both subcomponents of the process, as well as, ultimately, procedural control over how the process should be conducted. The amount of practice will need to be determined by the teacher while observing the apprentice becoming proficient in subcomponents. It would be critical to allow for enough practice so that operating on components is implicit and automatic. Once this has been accomplished, the apprentice would be able to allocate attentional resources to the higher-level, procedural demands of the task. At this point the teacher might begin to make comments about more explicit rules, verbalize about metaoperational procedures, or decide not to bring processes to the surface at an explicit level. The premature introduction of explicitly stated rules can have the effect of focusing attention on the learning and exercise of rules per se at the expense of attention to individual cases (Brooks, 1978). As such, the rule takes on an absolute, nonmodifiable authority. It is not likely to be modified due to the nature of the task to which it must be applied. Either an individual case fits the rule or it does not. The rule is destined to maintain its initial formulation rather than evolve into a higher-level structure. In contrast, individual cases can preserve the richness and variability of a concept or rule system. As such, they serve as prototypes or good examples that become analogues to be used in drawing inferences. The process of reasoning by analogy is an implicit one. It allows for a vagueness, a fuzziness that in turn allows for more flexible application. What reasoning by analogy or by any tacit process lacks in precision it gains in color and flavor, and, in its automaticity, has the potential to preserve capacity. Johnson-Laird (1985) warns us not to interfere with natural, tacit approaches to learning:

What we do know is that implicit inferences are so automatic that most people are unaware of making them. Like many skills, children must somehow pick up the ability in a wholly tacit way. This characteristic suggests that we must be especially careful that we do not unwittingly interfere with the normal acquisition of this skill, if we try to enhance it. The educational task is more akin to trying to promote the development of a child's native tongue than to giving explicit instruction (Johnson-Laird, 1985, p. 29).

The apprenticeship process has promised to be very effective. The cost in terms of time and patience, however, is considerable. In our experience it has been difficult to convince teachers as well as parents that "gains" attained too rapidly without a solid foundation may not lead to independent, generalized abilities.

Teachers in particular feel the need to demonstrate continual progress, onward and upward, and are hard to convince that they might consider taking each skill beyond mastery to automaticity before moving on. The gradual and systematic passage of control from teacher to child is a model that has worked in all cultures and for nearly all children during the developmental period. It promises to alleviate the problems of tenuous, easy-to-lose, situation-specific gains, which are so typical in children with handicaps to learning and are so resistant to generalization.

Ceding Cognitive Control to the Child

Another of the virtues of the apprenticeship relationship is its intimacy, which allows the teacher insight into the individual qualities of the learner. Whether the learner is in the role of apprentice or the more typical role of a learner in a larger, perhaps mainstreamed group, he or she arrives in the learning environment with a personal set of experiences and cognitive idiosyncrasies. These include not only the influences of the learner's dominant culture, familial background, and earlier schooling, but also those influences of the subculture in which children with handicaps evolve and live. We have indicated that children with handicaps inspire more directiveness, less responsivity, and fewer invitations for initiation than do nonhandicapped children. The transactions among initial child characteristics and experiences with others create the idiosyncrasies with which the child approaches or at least enters the learning situation. These need to be considered consciously in formulating effective instruction. Children with handicaps and those who have appeared vulnerable in the eyes of their caregivers or teachers inspire an instructional style in which the teacher controls and directs nearly all of the interaction. This may account at least partially for the confusion that learning-disabled and slow-learning children feel when they find themselves in groups of children with a similar lack of experience in self-direction. This dynamic is reported repeatedly and for a wide range of handicapping and risk conditions (Jones, 1980; Mahoney & Powell, 1986; Rocissano & Yatchmink, 1983). Nevertheless, it does not promise to be an optimal condition for promoting self-regulated learning. Although external regulation provides a comfort level and steers the child along the path of normative acquisitions, we have argued that neither comfort nor error-free advancement along a typical continuum constitutes a sound approach to learning. An important goal for instruction of handicapped learners will be to interfere in this cycle of external direction and internal receptivity at the expense of initiation, to pass control gradually to the child. The process is a delicate and frustrating one for both members of the dyad.

The child is used to receiving direction, to having most moves, thoughts, and decisions orchestrated, and is likely to be at a complete loss in its absence. The teacher is not likely to be given many gestures from the child to which he or she can respond. Without careful planning, the approach can end in a painfully non-productive waiting game. This can be avoided by using a model of the apprentice relationship and its potential for ceding gradual control to the child in a per-sonally and cognitively supportive context, rather than expecting the child to take charge immediately.

Adapting to the Child's Characteristics

Adults working with handicapped children will have a greater number of child initiations to which to respond if they will "reframe" the child's behaviors, recog-nizing some atypical behaviors as positive approaches to learning or problem solving. We have given some examples in Chapter 2 of how errors can be used in this way. More fundamentally, the very process that generated these errors should be valued as a reflection of the active, internal organization of the child and might be channeled in the effort to encourage active problem solving and metaprocedural control. So-called impulsive children who must say it now and loudly have some implicit awareness of the tenuousness of immediate and short-term memory as well as the usefulness of verbal rehearsal. Instead of telling the child to be quiet, a teacher might recognize this and use it, at first in its nonmodi-fied form, in the service of thinking and remembering. Once the process has been channeled into an efficient strategy, its usefulness and broader applicability might be made more explicit to the learner. At this point the child might be told that although this procedure is a good one, it is also disturbing to others. The child can be shown first how to speak softly, how to subvocalize, and perhaps will eventually be able to move his or her language completely inward.

The notion of good strategies for all learners might be modified to some degree. More to the point, the notion of bad strategies might be reevaluated. The conviction that "distractions" such as overextended elaborations, irrelevancies, or metacognitive wanderings are counterproductive has proved, in our research, to be not entirely valid. When learning-disabled children are left to their own devices, they do ponder the problem and select strategies spontaneously. Our findings suggest that successful strategic behavior in learning-disabled children is embedded in a context of one typically valued strategy, relevant connections, which has been the focus of much experimentation under the name of verbal mediation (Jensen & Rohwer, 1963). In the learning-disabled population, how-ever, this strategy is accompanied by other strategies, which also account for a respectable variance shared with success. In particular, overextended elabo-rations (see Chapter 3) and irrelevancies are likely to serve the purpose of main-taining arousal by keeping the stimuli relatively novel and thus increasing the quality and duration of attention (Fagan, 1982). Although this approach might seem indirect, it effectively avoids the need for internally controlled, focused, sustained, and vigilant attention for which many learning-disabled youngsters simply do not have the neurological or biochemical base (Kinsbourne, 1986). Instruction will need to consider the possibility that many strategies, even those with bad names, are potentially productive. We have been able to provide some evidence that mental wandering should be allowed and perhaps encouraged, at least up to a point and at least in learning-disabled children. This finding opens the possibility that there are additional strategies, previously judged as counter-productive, that might be equally beneficial in learning for some populations. Special education, it seems, will require continual efforts to understand the child's problem as much as its solution.

Metacognitive Interventions

In addition to generating effective strategies spontaneously, our learning-disabled population was capable of considerable metacognitive activity. They were more nearly like the gifted population than they were like any other group in their frequency of metacognitive strategy usage. The quality of metacognition in the two groups, however, was quite different. Whereas the gifted children tended to focus on weighing the virtues of various strategies and on what would need to be done to finish the job, the learning-disabled children spent their metacognitive awareness on concern for whether the task was easy or hard. The metacognitive function for them seemed to be to monitor task difficulty and success/failure rather than to direct or orchestrate problem-solving activity. Learning-disabled children seem to get stuck at this stage of the metacognitive process, perhaps due to lack of confidence and worry about whether they really would be able to muster the resources to meet the challenges of the task. For whatever reason, they rarely seem to reach the point of making a plan. Metacognitive interventions will need to be designed with this in mind. Those procedures that target increased monitoring and conscious awareness of the effectiveness of strategic behavior might be detrimental for children who are already monitoring to the point of being immobilized. Instead, for them the focus might be that suggested by Feuerstein and his colleagues: formulation of the plan for problem solving or learning. In fact, by asking the child not to solve but only to make a plan, the child's concerns about success and failure are obviated. Ironically, this procedure not only gains the cooperation and enthusiasm of most learning-disabled children, it also leads to quick and relatively painless successful solutions.

It is interesting to note that our learning-disabled children are more like the gifted in their use of strategies than like slow learners. This is surely due, in part, to our selection criteria and to the fact that the children were drawn mainly from suburban areas, which are associated with higher levels of socioeconomic status and enriched home environments. Not only were the learning-disabled children similar to gifted children in some respects, they used higher-level strategies than both the average and slow-learning children. Only the gifted surpassed them on this measure. This finding should not be news to those who work in the field. The definition of learning disabilities includes exactly this fact of average or above-average intelligence. Classroom teachers and parents express frustration about children whom they know to be bright, but who seem "unmotivated" or "oppositional." Despite our empirical, definitional, and intuitive awareness that children with learning disabilities have higher-level cognitive abilities, instruction is nearly uniformly based in procedures adopted from the education of persons with mental retardation, the main components of which are: make it simple, break it down, and avoid asking the learner to do the organizing, managing, and thinking. Ironically, our data suggest that learning-disabled children are already using higher-level strategies than those asked for in the context of this kind of instruction. Perhaps we cannot make it simple for them. The very fact that, by virtue of extreme discrepancies, they are taking the world in at two (or more) levels is complicating. We will need to instruct these children in the context of their own complexity. In addition, like many cognitively competent learners, learning-disabled children are motivated by a challenge that enhances their sense of competence, rather than by work that they regard as trivial, uninteresting, and failing to contribute to their sense of cognitive capability and self-worth. We have no prepackaged, neat prescriptions for how instruction should meet the paradox of the learning-disabled child. These findings tell us, however, that the solution is not likely to be found in models of instruction originally designed to meet the needs of mentally retarded or slow-learning children.

Instructional Needs of Slow Learners

In fact, the slow learners in our study present a quite different set of needs. Their spontaneous approaches are characterized as undifferentiated and global and as focusing on single aspects of the stimuli, such as descriptors of the pictures or labeling of only one of the pictures in the pair. What is markedly absent in their approach is the attempt to impose an association between the elements. Their strategies seem to reflect their tendency to attend to the surface features of the task at the expense of constructing or applying previously constructed, personalized mental models (Johnson-Laird, 1985). The most effective form of connection for slow learners was word play (*cup–cub*). It is likely that slow learners are lead into this form of association again by surface features, this time phonetic. Their group behavior was also characterized by concern with relatively superficial procedural matters, such as whose turn it would be next. The challenge for instruction of slow-learning children has been to induce deeper-level processing. Suggestions that have shown considerable promise are interrogative strategies (Borkowski & Cavanaugh, 1979), providing symmetry (Zeaman & House, 1963a, 1963b), accentuating invariant, critical features (Zeaman & House, 1963b); and other forms of organization external to the learner, possibly within the stimulus materials themselves (Spitz, 1966). All of these approaches have in common the reliance on externally placed organizing features. Since the slow learner is not likely to apply personal connections whether relevant, irrelevant, or overextended, it is important to program those connections for the child. One can imagine that this takes a great deal of planning, time in instruction, and monitoring of what has actually been noticed, processed, and stored. The effort is justified, at least theoretically, by the promise of establishing a larger and more richly integrated knowledge store, which in turn increases the likelihood that meaningful frames for organizing information might be invoked more spontaneously.

Despite our efforts to classify strategic behavior according to diagnostic category, the fact remains that each learner has his or her own distinct history of experiences, cognitive organization, and preferences for problem approach. Methods of instruction that are not firmly rooted in these as well as in general considerations for the instruction of learning-disabled versus slow-learning versus average children would surely miss the mark.

Mainstreaming

The distinct and idiosyncratic needs of each child with a handicap, then, require specialized, one-to-one instruction for the purposes of ongoing diagnosis as well as instruction designed to fit the learner. Since the advent of Public Law 94-142 and Section 504 of the Rehabilitation Act in 1973, however, mainstreaming has become a mandatory part of school life for the majority of special education students. Evaluations of the benefits of mainstreaming versus special education placement have produced mixed results (Budoff & Gottlieb, 1976; Carlberg & Kavale, 1980). Different categories of exceptional children do relatively well or less well in the regular class environment in various aspects of achievement or social adjustment. The problem is that most of the efforts at mainstreaming have taken a very limited and one-sided approach to the process. What we would like to suggest here is that the concept of mainstreaming is not merely the placement of handicapped students in a regular classroom, and that the success or failure of this procedure cannot be assessed by comparing, for example, the reading achievement of these children with that of children in a special class. From our point of view, mainstreaming is a philosophy based on a belief that it is in some fundamental way desirable for different types of children to interact together and learn many things from each other. The question is, then, how should classes be structured to meet the needs of both handicapped and average learners? In particular, how can the exceptional children be given exceptional opportunities within an ordinary classroom to take an active role, to learn from other students, and to gradually take over executive control of their learning?

It would seem axiomatic that not all children, even "average" children, learn at the same rate; some are generally slower, whereas others excel in one subject or another. This variability is even more marked if we include slow learners or children with specific learning disabilities in the group. One of the problems with many regular classrooms is that children are, in fact, all expected to learn in the same manner and at the same rate. Subject material is presented by the teacher, usually children are asked to give answers and are corrected if they are wrong, and, if they do not learn the concept or material within a set time, they are given a low grade. The teacher then passes on to the next topic. Too often the rationale is, if the child cannot learn regular class material, he or she does not belong in the regular class.

At the elementary level, the problem of diverse learning rates is often handled by dividing the children into ability groups within the classroom; the handicapped children usually make up the lowest group. Not only does this process underline the low status of the handicapped children, it does not address the true purpose of mainstreaming, which is to allow for the interaction of all the students. Another technique that is often employed is to preteach skills that are going to be covered in the mainstream. Again, this may help a child fit in with what is expected in terms of learning material at the same rate and in the same manner as the other children; the child adjusts, not the system.

In what ways, then, could the mainstream experience be reconceived to allow each child to learn to regulate his or her own learning according to personal needs? First, it must be recognized that the goals and objectives for exceptional students are individualized; it is not necessary for all students to proceed at the same rate for an experience to be educational. What is important is that the student makes progress in achieving his or her goals. Attempts to pass the student along the curriculum will actively interfere with the learning process of many students, as well as producing feelings of inadequacy. It could be argued that this is true of all students; it is especially critical for those with learning problems because of their more marked difficulties and history of failure.

We have placed considerable importance on the role of error making in problem solving, both in allowing the creative process of learning and understanding to proceed unhindered by the constraints of coming up with correct answers and in enabling teachers to understand how a student is thinking by noticing patterns among errors. By definition, a slow or different learner will produce more errors than a successful student if both are learning the same material. The successful student will understand what the teacher wants and give the desired answer. Whether this is the most productive method of teaching good students is another topic and is not our concern here. What is important is what happens to the student who does make a mistake. If the error is corrected without explanation, the student probably learns nothing and feels stupid. If, on the other hand, the reason for the error is analyzed to determine the basic cause of the lack of understanding, the teaching route can take a detour to create different learning experiences with the material. These points are most obvious in mathematics, where children frequently learn procedures by rote without understanding the reasons for what they are doing.

Another consideration involved in mainstreaming is the need to address the specific strengths and weaknesses of the individual student. Recommendations for a child with auditory attention deficits might include securing the child's attention, repetition of directions, preparing written summaries and study guides, and so on. On the other hand, a child with strong visual perceptual skills, whose difficulties lie in the area of language comprehension and expression, would need opportunities to interact with concrete materials and to create maps, diagrams, charts, and so forth whenever the opportunity arises. For such a child, the use of audiotapes would be counterproductive, whereas for a bright, verbal child with specific reading difficulties, such tapes could be a real asset in supplementing instruction. The need to implement all these special provisions can be seen as a burden by classroom teachers who have been trained in a "product" definition of education. Although some of this load can be relieved by consultation with special education teachers, the use of classroom aides, and so on, the true benefits of mainstreaming will only be seen when different goals and expectations are induced during teacher training. In any case, it should be clear by now that one of the prime considerations, regardless of the specific needs and adaptations involved, is the gradual, sensitive transition of responsibility and control from the teacher to the child.

Another very relevant topic that we have discussed at length is the effect of student interaction on learning. In Chapter 5 we presented some of the evidence that, in certain circumstances, cooperative learning can be beneficial to low-achieving students. On the other hand, the slow learners in our study, presented in Chapter 6, were so overwhelmed by the group situation that the quality of their memory strategies actually deteriorated. One obvious reason for this discrepancy is the homogeneity of our groups; the children were not able to reap the benefits of interaction with more successful learners. We are hoping to extend the study by examining the behavior and performance of mixed groups of low-achieving and average learners. Another possible explanation of our findings is that handicapped children are not exposed to the experience of working in groups or taught to do so productively. This requires quite sophisticated collaborative skills, such as decision making and conflict management, that do not occur spontaneously and may need to be taught directly before productive group work can occur.

In a discussion of mainstreaming and cooperative learning, Johnson and Johnson (1986) consider three of the most common problems occurring when handicapped students are mainstreamed into cooperative learning groups: the handicapped students being anxious or passively uninvolved, and the nonhandicapped students worrying about their grades being adversely affected. Some of the actions that can be taken to alleviate these concerns are explaining procedures, assigning structured roles according to a child's abilities and such that the group can only succeed if all members participate, pretraining on requisite collaborative skills, and using different criteria for success for the handicapped group members (such as improvement scores). Under these conditions, the mainstreaming experience can be fruitful for all students, not only those with educational handicaps.

Conclusion

As we look around at the real-world education of handicapped children, there seems to be an insurmountable chasm between the conclusions we have reached and what actually takes place in schools. Perhaps it is too fanciful to imagine that this gulf can be bridged and research evidence increasingly translated into class-room practice. We hope not. Certainly, our ideas are not value free, and we do not put them forward as such. We have raised some questions about the nature of learning in atypical children, without aiming to provide an easy solution. It is most likely that none exists. We are more interested in promoting critical discussion than in presenting a neat package of recommendations. What we do hope is that those involved in school administration and teacher education will become familiar with recent research into the learning and development of special children and seriously consider how this knowledge can be integrated into educational practice. Our challenge as educators is much like that of the children with whom we are concerned: understanding the problem and developing strategies for its solution. The problem of how each child learns best, most typically, or both, must be redefined and reconsidered with each new addition to the special education rolls.

Appendix A
Stimulus Materials

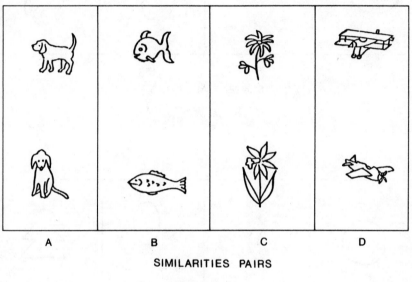

A   B   C   D

SIMILARITIES PAIRS

FIGURE A.1.

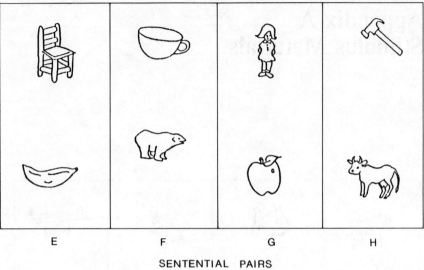

SENTENTIAL PAIRS

FIGURE A.2.

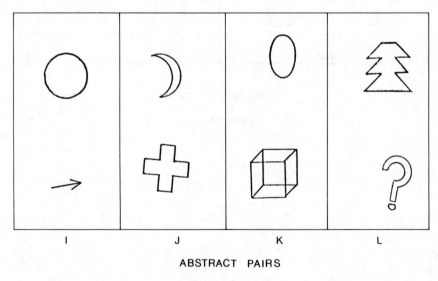

ABSTRACT PAIRS

FIGURE A.3.

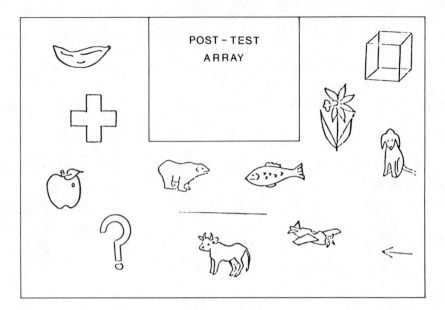

FIGURE A.4.

Appendix B
Strategy Scoring System

Labeling (L1 or L2): Naming of (1) one picture or (2) both pictures.

Example: A cup and a bear.

Labeling Question (LQ): Request for information about name of an item.

Example: What's that?

Information Question (IQ): Request for information other than names.

Example: Do we have to remember all of these?

Visual Description (VD1 and VD2): Description of the physical apsects of one or both pictures.

Example: This has a bit sticking out here.

Functional Description (FD1 and FD2): Description of a function or characteristic of one or both items.

Example: One's food and one's something you can sit on.

Functional Abstraction (FABS): Relationship based on an abstract connection or idea.

Example: I can remember because of going fishing.

Relevant Connection (CR): Relationship based on an interaction between two items.

Example: The girl can eat the apple.

Visual Connection (CV): Relation based on physical aspects of both pictures.

Example: The oval can fit in the box.

Labeling Similarity (LS): Statement of essential similarity of paired items.

Example: They're both flowers.

Relevant Similarities (SR): Relationship between pictures based on a specific similarity that aids recall.

Example: They both have fins.

Irrelevant Similarities (SIR): Relationship based on a similarity that is not specific to those pictures and does not necessarily aid recall.

Example: They're both little.

Visual Similarity (SV): Relationship based on the similarities in appearance of the two pictures.

Example: This part of the hammer looks like it's straight down like the cow's tail.

Functional Similarity (SF): Relationship based on similarity of function.

Example: You could use the cow and the hammer on a farm.

Similarity of Names (SN): Relationship based on similarity between names of both pictures.

Example: Ball and box both begin with "b."

Similarities and Differences (SRD): Recognition and description of difference between two otherwise similar items.

Example: These are both flowers and one has two long leaves and one has two little leaves.

Developed Differences (DD): Explanation of a difference between the two pictures.

Example: The cow's alive and the hammer isn't.

Visual Differences (DV): Explanation of a difference between physical aspects of the two pictures.

Example: That one has a round top and that one has a flat top.

Undeveloped Differences (DU): Statement of a difference without explanation.

Example: Because this one's different from that one.

Differences of Names (DN): Statement of a difference based on names of items.

Example: Remember cup with short "u" in the middle and bear with "e" in the middle.

Global Association (GA): Vague, unspecified statement of relationship.

Example: This one goes with this one.

Global Association of Names (GAN): Arbitrary connection between names of items.

Example: Remember "ch" for chair goes with "b" for banana.

Overextended Elaboration (OE): Long or involved story going beyond description or statement of relationship.

Example: You can sit on the chair and put the banana on your head or sit on the floor and put the chair on your head and the banana on top, or sit on the chair and eat the banana and put the peel on your head and then take a bath.

Irrelevant Comments (IRA): Off-task remarks.

Example: I'm going shopping this afternoon.

Irrelevant Comments (IRB): Irrelevant remarks related to the task.

Example: This is fun.

Meta-operations (MOA): Metacognitive comment about the task in general.

Example: The ones that are like each other are simple.

Meta-operations (MOB): Comment about strategies relating to a specific stimulus pair.

Example: That's not a good way to remember.

Word Play (WP): Attempt to establish a connection by using a play on words.

Example: A cub and a cup.

Elaboration (E): Development of a previously stated idea.

Example: A bull can ram into something and a hammer can nail into something. So they're both ramming something.

OK Question (OKQ): Attempt to obtain agreement about a given strategy.

Example: Do you think that's a good way to remember?

Finishing (FIN): Statement or question about whether enough discussion has taken place on a given card.

Personal Comment (P)

Example: I've got a dog like that.

Repetition (REP): Reference to the remark having already been made by one of the members of the group.

I was going to say that (ISAY)

Instruction (INS): Direction to the other members of the group.

Example: Put the card in the middle.

Turns: Comment about turn-taking.

Writing (W): Comment about the writing of the experimenters.

Beginning (B): Unfinished statement.

Agreement (A)

Disagreement (Z)

Don't Know or *No Response* (DK)

References

Acredolo, L.P. (1978). The development of spatial orientation in infancy. *Developmental Psychology, 14*, 224–234.

Allen, V.L., & Feldman, R.S. (1973). Learning through tutoring: Low-achieving children as tutors. *Journal of Experimental Education, 42*, 1–5.

Ames, G.J., & Murray, F.B. (1982). When two wrongs make a right: Promoting cognitive changes by social conflict. *Developmental Psychology, 18*, 894–897.

Amsel, A., & Roussel, J. (1952). Motivational properties of frustration: I. Effect on a running response of the addition of frustration to the motivational complex. *Journal of Exceptional Psychology, 43*, 363–368.

Appel, L.F., Cooper, R.G., McCarrell, N., Sims-Knight, J., Yussen, S.R., & Flavel, L.J.H. (1972). The development of the distinction between perceiving and memorizing. *Child Development, 43,* 1365–1381.

Arend, R., Gove, F., & Sroufe, L.A. (1979). Continuity of individual adaptation from infancy to kindergarten: A predictive study of ego-resiliency and curiosity in preschoolers. *Child Development, 50*, 950–999.

Ausubel, D.P., & Fitzgerald, D. (1962). Organizer, general background, and antecedent learning variables in sequential verbal learning. *Journal of Educational Psychology, 53*, 243–249.

Baillergon, R., & Graber, M. (1987). Where's the rabbit? 5-month old infants' representation of the height of a hidden object. *Cognitive Development, 2*(4), 375–392.

Bales, R.F. (1950). *Interaction process analysis: A method for the study of small groups.* Chicago: University of Chicago Press.

Bargh, J.A., & Schul, Y. (1980). On the cognitive benefits of teaching. *Journal of Educational Psychology, 72*, 593–604.

Barnard, K., Bee, H., & Hammond, M. (1984). Developmental changes in maternal interactions with term and preterm infants. *Infant Behavior and Development, 1*, 101–113.

Battelle Developmental Inventory. (1986). Allen, TX: DLM Teaching Resources.

Battig, W.F. (1975). Within-individual differences in cognitive processes. In R.L. Solso (Ed.), *Information processing and cognition* (pp. 195–228). Hillsdale, NJ: Lawrence Erlbaum Associates.

Bauer, R.H. (1977). Memory processes in children with learning disabilities: Evidence for deficient rehearsal. *Journal of Experimental Child Psychology, 24*, 415–430.

Bearison, D.J. (1982). New directions in studies of social interaction and cognitive growth. In F. Seratica (Ed.), *Social cognition, context, and social behavior: A developmental perspective* (pp. 199–221). New York: Guilford Press.

146   References

Beilin, H. (1965). Learning and operational convergence in logical thought development. *Journal of Experimental Child Psychology, 2,* 411–420.

Belmont, J.M., & Butterfield, E.C. (1971). Learning strategies as determinants of memory deficiencies. *Cognitive Psychology, 2,* 411–420.

Belmont, J.M., & Butterfield, E.C. (1977). The instructional approach to developmental cognitive research. In R.V. Kail, Jr. & J.W. Hagen (Eds.), *Perspectives on the development of memory and cognition.* Hillsdale, NJ: Lawrence Erlbaum Associates.

Belmont, J.M., Ferretti, R.P., & Mitchell, D.W. (1982). Memorizing: A test of untrained mildly mentally retarded children's problem solving. *American Journal of Mental Deficiency, 87*(2), 197–210.

Belsky, J., Garduque, L., & Hrncir, E. (1984). Assessing performance competence and executive capacity in infant play: Relations to home environment and security of attachment. *Developmental Psychology, 20*(3), 406–417.

Bem, D.J., & McConnell, H.K. (1970). Testing the self-perception explanation of dissonance phenomena: On the salience of premanipulation attitudes. *Journal of Personality and Social Psychology, 14,* 23–31.

Berndt, T.J. (1981). Relations between social cognition, nonsocial cognition, and social behavior: The case of friendship. In J.H. Flavell & L. Ross (Eds.), *Social Cognitive Development.* Cambridge, MA: Cambridge University Press.

Bernstein, B. (1962). Social structure, language and learning. *Language and Speech, 5,* 31–48.

Bertrand, J.P. (1987). *A comparison of requests for information used by adults in a referential communication task with preschoolers.* Masters Thesis, University of Connecticut, Storrs.

Blankenship, C.S. (1978). Remediating systematic inversion errors in subtraction through the use of demonstration and feedback. *Learning Disability Quarterly, 1,* 12–22.

Boder, E. (1971). Developmental dyslexia: A diagnostic screening procedure based on three characteristic patterns of reading and spelling. *Journal of Learning Disabilities, 4,* 297–342.

Borkowski, J.G., & Cavanaugh, J.C. (1979). Maintenance and generalization of skills and strategies by the retarded. In N.R. Ellis (Ed.), *Handbook of mental deficiency, psychological theory, and research.* Hillsdale, NJ: Lawrence Erlbaum Associates.

Borkowski, J.G., Levers, S.R., & Gruenenfleder, T.M. (1976). Transfer of mediational strategies in children: The role of activity and awareness during strategy acquisition. *Child Development, 47,* 779–786.

Boucher, C.R. (1984). Pragmatics: The verbal language of learning disabled and nondisabled boys. *Learning Disability Quarterly, 7,* 271–286.

Bourne, L.E., & O'Banion, K. (1971). Conceptual rule learning and chronological age. *Developmental Psychology, 5*(3), 200–205.

Bower, T.G.R. (1964). Discrimination of depth in premotor infants. *Psychonomic Science, 1,* 368.

Bowerman, M. (1982). Starting to talk worse: Clues to language acquisition from children's late speech errors. In S. Strauss (Ed.), *U-shaped behavioral growth.* New York: Academic Press.

Bransford, J.C. (1979). *Human cognition: Learning, understanding, and remembering.* Belmont, CA: Wadsworth.

Bransford, J.C., Franks, J.J., Morris, C.D., & Stein, B.S. (1979). Some general constraints on learning and memory research. In L.S. Cermak & F.I.M. Craik (Eds.), *Levels of processing in human memory.* Hillsdale, NJ: Lawrence Erlbaum Associates.

Bray, N.W. (1979). Strategy production in the retarded. In N.R.Ellis (Ed.), *Handbook of mental deficiency, psychological theory, and research* (pp. 629–726). Hillsdale, NJ: Lawrence Erlbaum Associates.

Brooks, L. (1978). Nonanalytic concept formation and memory for instances. In E. Rosch & B.B. Hoyd (Eds.), *Cognition and categorization*. Hillsdale, NJ: Lawrence Erlbaum Associates.

Brown, A.L. (1975). The development of memory: Knowing, knowing about knowing, and knowing how to know. In H.W. Reese (Ed.), *Advances in child development and behavior* (Vol. 10). New York: Academic Press.

Brown, A.L. (1978). Knowing when, where, and how to remember: A problem of metacognition. In R. Glaser (Ed.), *Advances in instructional psychology* (Vol. 1, pp. 77–163). Hillsdale, NJ: Lawrence Erlbaum Associates.

Brown, A.L. (1979). Theories of memory and the problems of development, activity, growth, and knowledge. In L.S. Cermak & F.I.M. Craik (Eds.), *Levels of processing in human memory*. Hillsadle, NJ: Lawrence Erlbaum Associates.

Brown, A.L. (1982). Learning and development: The problem of compatibility, access, and induction. *Human Development, 25*, 89–115.

Brown, A.L., Bransford, J., Ferrara, R., & Campione, J. (1983). Learning, remembering, and understanding. In P.H. Mussen (Ed.), *Handbook of child psychology* (Vol. III, pp. 77–166). New York: John Wiley & Sons.

Brown, A.L., & Ferrara, R. (1985). Diagnosing the zone of proximal development. In J.V. Wertsch (Ed.), *Culture, communication, and cognition: Vygotskian perspectives*. New York: Cambridge University Press.

Brown, A.L., & French, L.A. (1979). The zone of potential development: Implications for intelligence testing in the year 2000. *Intelligence, 3*, 255–273.

Brown, A.L., Palincsar, A.S., & Armbruster, B.B. (1984). Instructing comprehension-fostering activities in interactive learning situations. In H. Mandal, N.L. Stein, & T. Trabasso (Eds.), *Learning and comprehension of text*. Hillsdale, NJ: Lawrence Erlbaum Associates.

Brown, A.L., & Smiley, S.S. (1977). Rating the importance of structural units of prose passages: A problem of metacognition. *Child Development, 48*, 1–8.

Brown, R. (1958). *Words and things*. Glencoe, IL: Free Press.

Bruner, J.S. (1973). Organization of early skilled action. *Child Development, 44*, 92–96.

Bruner, J.S. (1985). On teaching thinking: An afterthought. In S. Chipman, J. Segal, & R. Glaser (Eds.), *Thinking and learning skills*. Hillside, NJ: Lawrence Erlbaum Associates.

Bruner, J.S., Goodnow, J.J., & Austin, G.A. (1956). *A study of thinking*. New York: John Wiley & Sons.

Bruner, J.S., Olver, R.R., & Greenfield, P.M. (1966). *Studies in cognitive growth*. New York: John Wiley & Sons.

Bryan, T. (1986). Personality and situational factors in learning disabilities. In G. Paulides & D.F. Fisher (Eds.), *Dyslexia, its neuropsychology and treatment*. New York: John Wiley & Sons.

Bryan, T.H., & Bryan, J.H. (1978). Social interactions of learning disabled children. *Learning Disability Quarterly, 1*, 33–38.

Budoff, M., & Corman, L. (1976). Effectiveness of a learning potential procedure in improving problem-solving skills of retarded and nonretarded children. *American Journal of Mental Deficiency, 81*(3), 260–264.

Budoff, M., & Gottlieb, J. (1976). Special class EMR children mainstreamed: A study of aptitude (learning potential) × treatment interaction. *American Journal of Mental Deficiency, 81,* 1–11.

Bugelski, B.R., Kidd, E., & Segmen, J. (1968). Images as mediators in one-trial paired-associate learning. *Journal of Experimental Psychology, 76,* 69–73.

Burger, A.L., Blackman, L.S., & Clark, H.S. (1981). Generalization of verbal abstraction strategies by EMR children and adolescents. *American Journal of Mental Deficiency, 85*(6), 611–618.

Burger, A.L., Blackman, L.S., Clark, H.S., & Gordon, R. (1982). *The far generalization of visual analogies strategies in impulsive and reflective EMRs.* Paper presented at the Gatlinburg Conference, Gatlinburg, TN.

Burns, S., Haywood, C., Cox, J., Brooks, P., Green, K., Ransom, O., Goodroe, E., & Willis, E. (1983). *Let's think about it: A cognitive curriculum for young children.* Paper presented at the Division of Early Childhood Education Conference, Washington, DC.

Butterfield, E.C., Wambold, C., & Belmont, J.M. (1973). On the theory and practice of improving short-term memory. *American Journal of Mental Deficiency, 77,* 654–669.

Campione, J.C., & Brown, A.L. (1974). The effects of contextual changes and degree of component mastery on transfer of training. In H.W. Reese (Ed.), *Advances in child development and behavior* (Vol. 9). New York: Academic Press.

Campione, J.S., Brown, A.L., & Ferrara, R.A. (1982). Mental retardation and intelligence. In R.J. Sternberg (Ed.), *Handbook of human intelligence.* New York: Cambridge University Press.

Cardoso-Martins, C., Mervis, C.B., & Mervis, C.A. (1985). Early vocabulary acquisitions in Down's syndrome. *American Journal of Mental Deficiency, 90*(2), 177–184.

Carlberg, C., & Kavale, K. (1980). The efficacy of special versus regular class placement for exceptional children: A meta-analysis. *Journal of Special Education, 14,* 295–309.

Caron, A., & Caron, R. (1981). Processing of relational information as an index of infant risk. In S. Friedman & M. Sigman (Eds.), *Preterm birth and psychological development.* New York: Academic Press.

Case, R. (1978). Piaget and beyond: Toward a developmentally based theory and technology of instruction. In R. Glaser (Ed.), *Advances in instructional psychology* (Vol. 1, pp. 167–228). Hillsdale, NJ: Lawrence Erlbaum Associates.

Case, R. (1985). A developmentally based approach to the problem of instructional design. In S. Chipman, J. Segal, & R. Glaser (Eds.), *Thinking and learning skills* (Vol. 2, pp. 545–562). Hillsdale, NJ: Lawrence Erlbaum Associates.

Cavanaugh, J.C., & Borkowski, J.G. (1980). Searching for metamemory–memory connections: A developmental study. *Developmental Psychology, 16,* 441–453.

Cawley, J.F. (1985). *Cognitive strategies and mathematics.* Rockville, MD: Aspen Publishing.

Ceci, S.J., & Bronfenbrenner, V. (1985). Don't forget to take the cupcakes out of the oven: Prospective memory, strategic time-monitoring and context. *Child Development, 56*(1), 152–164.

Charlesworth, W.R. (1976). Human intelligence as adaptation: An ethological approach. In L.B. Resnick (Ed.), *The nature of intelligence* (pp. 147–168). New York: John Wiley & Sons.

Cherkes-Julkowski, M. (1985). Metacognitive considerations in mathematics instruction for the learning disabled. In J.F. Cawley (Ed.), *Cognitive strategies and mathematics for the learning disabled* (pp. 99–116). Rockville, MD: Aspen Publishing.

Cherkes-Julkowski, M., Bertrand, J., Roth, D., & Bradley, K. (1987). *Mothers as teachers of their preterm and full term children at age 20 months*. Paper given at Gatlinburg Conference, Gatlinburg, TN.

Cherkes-Julkowski, M., Davis, L., Fimian, M., Gertner, N., McGuire, J., Norlander, K., Okolo, C., & Zoback, M. (1986). Encouraging flexible strategy usage in handicapped learners. In J.M. Berg (Ed.), *Science and service in mental retardation* (pp. 189–196). London: Methuen.

Cherkes-Julkowski, M., Foley, G., Davis, L., Marrion, G., & Roth, D. (1985). *Development of preterm and full term infant dyads: A preliminary report*. Paper presented at the Fourth Annual National Clinical Infant Studies Conference, Washington, DC.

Cherkes-Julkowski, M., Gertner, N., & Norlander, K. (1986). Differences in cognitive processes among handicapped and average children: A group learning approach. *Journal of Learning Disabilities, 19*(7), 438–445.

Chi, M. (1985). Interactive roles of knowledge and strategies in the development of organized sorting and recall. In S. Chipman, J. Segal, & R. Glaser (Eds.), *Thinking and learning skills* (Vol. 2, pp. 457–484). Hillsdale, NJ: Lawrence Erlbaum Associates.

Chi, M.T.H., & Koeske, R.D. (1978). Knowledge structure and memory development. In R. Siegler (Ed.), *Children's thinking: What develops?* Hillsdale, NJ: Lawrence Erlbaum Associates.

Chi, M.T.H. (1983). Network representation of a child's dinosaur knowledge. *Developmental Psychology, 19*, 29–39.

Cohen, Y.A. (1971). The shaping of men's minds: Adaptations to the imperatives of culture. In M.L. Wax, S. Diamond, & F.O. Gearing (Eds.), *Anthropological perspectives on education*. New York: Basic Books.

Cole, M., & Scribner, S. (1975). Theorizing about socialization of cognition. *Ethos, 3*, 250–268.

Cole, M., & Scribner, S. (1984). *Culture and thought: A psychological introduction*. New York: John Wiley & Sons.

Cooper, L.A., & Shepard, R.N. (1973). Chronometric studies of the rotation of mental images. In W.G. Chase (Ed.), *Visual information processing*. New York: Academic Press.

Craik, F.I.M., & Lockhart, R.S. (1972). Levels of processing: A framework for memory research. *Journal of Verbal Learning and Verbal Behavior, 11*, 671–684.

Dallago, M.L., & Moely, B.E. (1980). Free recall in boys of normal and poor reading levels as a function of task manipulation. *Journal of Experimental Child Psychology, 30*, 62–78.

Damon, W. (1979). Why study social–cognitive development? *Human Development, 22*, 206–211.

Dansereau, D.F., Collins, K.W., McDonald, B.A., Holley, C.D., Garland, J.C., Diekhoff, G.M., & Evans, S.H. (1979). Development and evaluation of an effective learning strategy program. *Journal of Educational Psychology, 7*, 64–73.

Dawson, M.M., Hallahan, D.P., Reeve, R.E., & Ball, D.W. (1980). The effect of reinforcement and verbal rehearsal on selective attention in learning disabled children. *Journal of Abnormal Child Psychology, 8*, 133–144.

Day, J.D., French, L.A., & Hall, L.K. (1985). Social influences on cognitive development. In D.L. Forrest-Pressley, G.E. MacKinnon, & T.G. Waller (Eds.), *Metacognition, cognition, and human performance* (Vol. 1, pp. 33–56). New York: Academic Press.

DeLoache, J., Sugarman, S., & Brown, A. (1981, April). *Self-correction strategies in early cognitive development*. Paper presented at the meeting of the Society for Research in Child Development, Boston.

DeLoache, J.S. (1980). Naturalistic studies of memory for object location in very young children. *New Directions for Child Development, 10*, 17–32.

DeLoache, J.S. (1984). Oh where, Oh where: Memory-based searching by very young children. In C. Sophian (Ed.), *Origins of cognitive skills* pp. 57–80). Hillsdale, NJ: Lawrence Erlbaum Associates.

DeLoache, J.S., & Brown, A. (1983). Very young children's memory for location of objects in a large-scale environment. *Child Development, 54*, 888–897.

Delquadri, J., Greenwood, C.R., Stretton, K., & Hall, R.V. (1983). The peer tutoring game: A classroom procedure for increasing opportunity to respond and spelling performance. *Education and Treatment of Children, 6*, 225–239.

De Meuron, M., & Auerswald, E.A. (1969). Cognition and social adaptation. *American Journal of Orthopsychiatry, 39*, 57–67.

Denckla, M.B. (1972). Clinical syndromes in learning disabilities: The case for "Splitting" vs "Lumping." *Journal of Learning Disabilities, 5*, 401–406.

Denney, N.W., & Turner, M.C. (1979). Facilitating cognitive performance in children: A comparison of strategy modeling and strategy modeling with overt self-verbalization. *Journal of Experimental Child Psychology, 28*, 119–131.

Doise, W., & Mugny, G. (1979). Individual and collective conflicts of centrations in cognitive development. *European Journal of Social Psychology, 9*, 105–108.

Doise, W., Mugny, G., & Perret-Clermont, A.N. (1976). Social interaction and cognitive development: Further evidence. *European Journal of Social Psychology, 6*, 245–247.

Donahue, M. (1986). Linguistic and communicative development in learning disabled children. In S.J. Ceci (Ed.), *Handbook of cognitive, social, and neuropsychological aspects of learning disabilities*. Hillsdale, NJ: Lawrence Erlbaum Associates.

Donahue, M., Bryan, T., & Pearl, R. (1980, June). *Learning disabled children's conversational strategies in a decision making task with peers*. Paper presented at the First Symposium on Research in Child Language Disorders, University of Wisconsin, Madison.

Donald, J. (1982). *The development of knowledge structures*. Paper presented at the American Educational Research Association, New York.

Dudley-Marling, C.C. (1985). The pragmatic skills of learning disabled children: A review. *Journal of Learning Disabilities, 4*, 193–199.

Dudley-Marling, C.C., & Edmiaston, R. (1985). The social status of learning disabled children and adolescents: A review. *Learning Disability Quarterly, 8*, 189–210.

Dunst, C.J. (1980). *A clinical and educational manual for use with the Uzgiris–Hunt Scales of Infant Development*. Baltimore: University Park Press.

Durkin, H.E. (1937). Trial-and-error, gradual analysis and sudden reorganization: An experimental study of problem solving. *Archives of Psychology, 210*.

Durling, R., & Schick, C. (1976). Concept attainment by pairs and individuals as a function of vocalization. *Journal of Educational Psychology, 68*, 83–91.

Dweck, C. (1987, April). Children's Theories of intelligence: Implications for Motivation and learning. Invited Address, AERA Annual Meeting, Washington, DC.

Elliott, J.L., & Gentile, J.R. (1986). The efficacy of a mnemonic technique for learning disabled and nondisabled adolescents. *Journal of Learning Disabilities, 19*, 237–241.

Engle, R.W., & Nagle, R.J. (1979). Strategy training and semantic encoding in mildly retarded children. *Intelligence, 3*, 17–30.

Engle, R.W., Nagle, R.J., & Dick, M. (1980). Maintenance and generalization of a semantic rehearsal strategy in educable mentally retarded children. *Journal of Experimental Child Psychology, 30*, 438–454.

Ennis, R.H. (1976). An alternative to Piaget's conceptualization of logical competence. *Child Development, 47*, 903–919.

Ericsson, K.A., & Simon, H.A. (1980). Verbal reports as data. *Psychological Review, 87*, 215–251.

Fagan, J. (1982). Infant memory. In T. Field, A. Huston, H. Quay, L. Troll, & G. Finley (Eds.), *Review of human development* (pp. 79–92). New York: John Wiley & Sons.

Fantz, R.L. (1961). The origin of form perception. *Scientific American, 204*, 66–72.

Feagans, L. (1980). *Communication skills in learning disabled children*. Paper presented at the Annual Meeting of the National Convention of the Association for Children with Learning Disabilities, Milwaukee, WI.

Feuerstein, R. (1979). The dynamic assessment of retarded performers. *The learning potential assessment device, theory, instruments, and techniques*. Baltimore: University Park Press.

Feuerstein, R. (1980). *Instrumental enrichment: An intervention program for cognitive modifiability*. Baltimore: University Park Press.

Feuerstein, R., Jensen, M., Hoffman, M., & Rand, Y. (1985). Instrumental enrichment, an intervention program for structural cognitive modifiability. In J.W. Segal, S.F. Chipman, & R. Glaser (Eds.), *Thinking and learning skills* (Vol. 1, pp. 43–82). Hillsdale, NJ: Lawrence Erlbaum Associates.

Field, T. (1977). Effects of early separation, interactive deficits, and experimental manipulations on infant–mother face-to-face interaction. *Child Development, 11*, 42–49.

Flavell, J.H. (1963). The developmental psychology of Jean Piaget. Princeton, NJ: Van Nostrand.

Flavell, J.H. (1970). Developmental studies of mediated memory. In H.W. Reese & L.P. Lipsitt (Eds.), *Advances in child development and behavior* (Vol. 5). New York, Academic Press.

Flavell, J.H. (1977). *Cognitive development*. Englewood Cliffs, NJ: Prentice-Hall.

Fodor, J.A. (1975). *The language of thought*. Cambridge, MA: Harvard University Press.

Fodor, J.A. (1981). *Representation*. Cambridge MA: MIT Press.

Foley, G., & Hobin, M. (1981). *Attachment–Separation–Individuation Scale*. Reading, PA: Albright College.

Forman, E., & Cazden, C.B. (1985). Exploring Vygotskian perspectives in education: The cognitive value of peer interaction. In J.V. Wertsch (Ed.), *Culture, communication, and cognition: Vygotskian perspectives* (pp. 323–347). New York: Cambridge University Press.

Fraiberg, S. (1977). *Insights from the blind*. New York: Basic Books.

Frankenburg, W.K., Dodds, J., & Fandal, A. (1975). *Denver Developmental Screening Test*. Denver: LADOCA Project and Publishing Foundation.

Furuno, S., O'Reilly, K.A., Hosaka, C.M., Inatsuka, T.T., Allman, T.L., & Zeisloft, B. (1979). *Hawaii early learning profile and activity guide*. Palo Alto, CA: VORT Corporation.

Gardner, W., & Rogoff, B. (1982). The role of instruction in memory development: Some methodological choices. *Quarterly Newsletter of the Laboratory of Comparative Human Cognition, 4*, 6–12.

Gelabert, A.R., Torgesen, J.K., Dice, C., & Murphy, H. (1980). The effects of situational variables on the use of rehearsal by first grade children. *Child Development, 51*(3), 902–905.

Gelman, R., & Spelke, R. (1981). The development of thoughts about animate and inanimate objects: Implications for research on social cognition. In J.H. Flavell & L. Ross (Eds.), *Social cognitive development: Frontiers and possible futures.* New York: Cambridge University Press.

Gerjuoy, I.R., & Spitz, H.H. (1966). Associative clustering in free recall: Intellectual and developmental variables. *American Journal of Mental Deficiency, 70,* 918-927.

Gesell, A., & Amatruda, C.S. (1947). *Developmental diagnosis.* New York: Harper & Row.

Gesell, A.L. (1940). *Wolf child and human child.* New York: Harper & Row.

Ghiselin, B. (1952). *The creative process.* New York: Mentor.

Gibson, E., & Rader, N. (1979). Attention. In G. Hall & M. Lewis (Eds.), *Attention and cognitive development.* New York: Plenum.

Glidden, L.M. (1979). Training of learning and memory in retarded persons: Strategies, techniques, and teaching tools. In N.R. Ellis (Eds.), *Handbook of mental deficiency, psychological theory, and research.* Hillsdale, NJ: Lawrence Erlbaum Associates.

Glidden, L.M., Bilsky, L.H., Mar, H.H., Judd, T.P., & Warner, D.A. (1983). Semantic processing can facilitate free recall in mildly retarded adolescents. *Journal of Experimental Child Psychology, 36,* 510-532.

Glidden, L.M., Bilsky, L.H., & Pawelski, C. (1977). Sentence mediation and stimulus blocking in free recall. *American Journal of Mental Deficiency, 82,* 84-90.

Glidden, L.M., & Warner, D.A. (1983). Semantic processing and recall improvement of EMR adolescents. *American Journal of Mental Deficiency, 88,* 96-105.

Goethals, G.R., & Reckman, R.F. (1973). The perception of consistency in attitudes. *Journal of Experimental and Social Psychology, 9,* 491-501.

Goldberg, S., & DeVitto, B. (1983). *Born too soon: Preterm birth and early development.* San Francisco: W.H. Freeman.

Goldman-Rakic, P.S. (1987). Development of cortical circuitry and cognitive function. *Child Development, 58*(3), 601-622.

Goodnow, J.J. (1976). The nature of intelligent behavior: Questions raised by cross-cultural studies. In L. B. Resnick (Ed.), *The nature of intelligence* (pp. 169-188). New York: John Wiley & Sons.

Gordon, D.A., & Baumeister, A.A. (1971). The use of verbal mediation in the retarded as a function of developmental level and response availability. *Journal of Experimental Child Psychology, 12,* 95-105.

Greenfield, P.M., & Bruner, J.S. (1969). Culture and cognitive growth. In D.A. Goslin (Ed.), *Handbook of socialization theory and research.* New York: Rand McNally.

Greenough, W.T., Black, J.E., & Wallace, C.S. (1987). Experience and brain development. *Child Development, 58(3),* 539-559.

Greenwood, C.R., Delquadri, J., & Hall, R.V. (1984). Opportunity to respond and student academic performance. In W.L. Heward, T.E. Heron, J. Trap-Porter, & D.S. Hill (Eds.), *Focus on behavior analysis in education* (pp. 58-88). Columbus, OH: Charles Merrill.

Gronlund, N. (1976). *Measurement and evaluation in teaching* (3rd ed.). New York: Macmillan.

Hagen, J.W., & Kingsley, P.R. (1968). Labeling effects in short-term memory. *Child Development, 39,* 113-121.

Haines, D.J., & Torgesen, J.K. (1979). The effects of incentives on rehearsal and short-term memory in children with reading problems. *Learning Disability Quarterly, 2,* 48-55.

Hall, L.K., & Day, J.D. (1982). *A comparison of the zone of proximal development in learning disabled, mentally retarded, and normal children.* Paper presented at the meeting of the American Educational Research Association, New York.

Hall, R.V., Delquadri, J., Greenwood, C.R., & Thurston, L. (1982). The importance of opportunity to respond in children's academic success. In E. Edgar, N. Haring, J. Jenkins, & C. Pious (Eds.), *Mentally handicapped children: Education and training* (pp. 107–140. Baltimore: University Park Press.

Hallahan, D.P., Tarver, S.G., Kauffman, J.M., & Graybeal, N.L. (1979). Selective attention abilities of learning disabled children under reinforcement and response cost. *Journal of Learning Disabilities, 11,* 42–51.

Hammill, D.D. (1985). *Detroit Test of Learning Aptitude*-2. Austin, TX: Pro-Ed.

Harris, J.E. (1980). Memory aids people use: Two interview studies. *Memory and cognition, 8,* 31–38.

Haskins, R., & McKinney, J.D. (1976). Relative effects of response tempo and accuracy on problem solving and academic achievement. *Child Development, 47,* 690–696.

Haywood, C.A. (1977). Cognitive approach to the education of retarded children. *Peabody Journal of Education, 54,* 110–116.

Held, R., & Hein, A. (1963). Movement produced stimulation in the development of visually guided behavior. *Journal of Comparative and Physiological Psychology, 81,* 394–398.

Hess, R.D., Holloway, S.D., Dickson, W.P., & Price, G.G. (1984). Maternal variables as predictors of children's school readiness and later achievement in vocabulary and mathematics in 6th grade. *Child Development, 55,* 1902–1912.

Hess, R.D., & Shipman, V. (1965). Early experience and the socialization of cognitive modes in children. *Child Development, 36,* 869–886.

Hodapp, R., Goldfield, E., & Boyatzis, J. (1984). The use and effectiveness of maternal scaffolding in mother–infant games. *Child Development, 55,* 772–781.

Howe, M.L., Brainerd, C.J., & Kingma, J. (1985). Storage–retrieval process of normal and learning disabled children. *A Stages-of-Learning Analysis of Picture–Word Effects, 56(5),* 1120–1133.

Hudgins, B. (1960). Effects of group experience on individual problem solving. *Journal of Educational Psychology, 51,* 37–42.

Hundeide, K. (1985). The tacit background of children's judgements. In J.V. Wertsch (Ed.), *Culture, communication, and cognition: Vygotskian perspectives* (pp. 306–322). New York: Cambridge University Press.

Hupp, S.C., Conroy, M., & Able, H. (1986). Designing instructional programs to facilitate generalization of object categories by young handicapped children. *Journal of the Division for Early Childhood, 10(2),* 149–155.

Jacoby, L.L., Bartz, W.H., & Evans, J.D. (1978). A functional approach to levels of processing. *Journal of Experimental Psychology: Human learning and Memory, 4,* 331–346.

Jenkins, J.J. (1979). Four points to remember: A tetrahedral model and memory experiments. In L.S. Cermak & F.I.M. Craik (Eds.), *Levels of processing in human memory.* Hillsdale, NJ: Lawrence Erlbaum Associates.

Jenkins, J.R., Mayall, U.R., Peschka, C.M., & Henkins, L.M. (1974). Comparing small group and tutorial instruction in resource rooms. *Exceptional Children, 40,* 245–250.

Jensen, A.R., & Rohwer, W.D. (1963). The effect of verbal mediation on the learning and retention of paired-associates by retarded adults. *American Journal of Mental Deficiency, 68,* 80–84.

John, V. (1963). The intellectual development of slum children: Some preliminary findings. *American Journal of Orthopsychiatry, 33*, 813–822.

Johnson, D., Maruyama, G., Johnson, R., Nelson, D., & Skon, L. (1981). The effects of cooperative, competitive, and individualistic goal structures on achievement: A meta-analysis. *Psychological Bulletin, 9*, 47–62.

Johnson, D.W. (1979). Student–student interaction: The neglected variable in education. *Educational Researcher, 10*, 5–10.

Johnson, D.W., & Johnson, R.T. (1986). Mainstreaming and cooperative learning strategies. *Exceptional Children, 52*, 553–561.

Johnson-Laird, P.N. (1983). *Mental models.* Cambridge, MA: Harvard University Press.

Johnson-Laird, P.N. (1985). Logical thinking: Does it occur in daily life? Can it be taught? In S. Chipman, J. Segal, & R. Glaser (Eds.), *Thinking and learning skills* (Vol. 2, pp. 293–318). Hillsdale, NJ: Lawrence Erlbaum Associates.

Jones, O.H. (1980). Prelinguistic communication skills in Down's syndrome and normal infants. In T. Field, S. Goldberg, D. Stern, & A.M. Sostek (Eds.), *High-risk infants and children: Adult and peer interactions* (pp. 205–226). New York: Academic Press.

Jordan, E., Ackerman, J., & Wicker, F.W. (1977). Provided visual mediators, imagery instructions, and concreteness in paired associate learning. *Bulletin of the Psychonomic Society, 9*, 124–126.

Kane, B.J., & Alley, G.R. (1980). A peer-tutored, instructional management program in computational mathematics for incarcerated learning disabled juvenile delinquents. *Journal of Learning Disabilities, 13*, 39–42.

Karmiloff-Smith, A. (1979). A problem-solving construction and representations of closed railway circuits. *Archives of Psychology, 47*, 37–59.

Karmiloff-Smith, A. (1981). Getting developmental differences or studying child development. *Cognition, 10*, 151–158.

Karmiloff-Smith, A., & Inhelder, B. (1974/75). If you want to get ahead, get a theory. *Cognition, 3*, 195–212.

Kaufman, A.S., & Kaufman, N.L. (1983). *Kaufman Assessment Battery for Children.* Circle Pines, MN: American Guidance Service.

Kaufman, A.S., & McLean, J.E. (1986). K-ABC/WISC-R factor analysis for a learning disabled population. *Journal of Learning Disabilities, 19(3)*, 145–153.

Kaye, K. (1982a). Organism, apprentice, and person. In E.Z. Tronick (Ed.), *Social interchange in infancy.* Baltimore: University Park Press.

Kaye, K. (1982b). *The mental and social life of babies, how parents create persons.* Chicago: University of Chicago Press.

Kellas, G., Ashcraft, M.H., & Johnson, S. (1973). Rehearsal processes in the short-term memory performance of mildly retarded adults. *American Journal of Mental Deficiency, 77*, 670–679.

King, R.T. (1982). Learning from a PAL. *The Reading Teacher, 35*, 682–685.

Kinsbourne, M. (1986). Models of dyslexia and its subtypes. In G.T. Paulidis & D.F. Fisher (Eds.), *Dyslexia: Its neuropsychology and treatment* (pp. 165–180). New York: John Wiley & Sons.

Knifong, J.D. (1974). Logical abilities of young children—Two styles of approach. *Child Development, 45*, 78–83.

Knight-Arest, I. (1984). Communicative effectiveness of learning disabled and normally achieving 10 to 13 year old boys. *Learning Disability Quarterly, 7*, 237–245.

Kohlberg, L. (1958). *The development of modes of moral thinking and choice in years 10 to 16.* Unpublished doctoral dissertation, University of Chicago.

Kol'tsova, V.A. (1978). Experimental study of cognitive activity in communication (with special reference to concept formation). *Soviet Psychology, 17*, 23–38.

Krakow, J., & Kopp, C. (1983). The effect of developmental delays on sustained attention in young children. *Child Development, 54*, 1143–1155.

Kramer, J.J., & Engle, R.W. (1981). Teaching awareness of strategic behavior in combination with strategy training: Effects on children's memory performance. *Journal of Experimental Child Psychology, 32*, 513–530.

Kreutzer, M.A., Leonard, C., & Flavell, J.H. (1975). An interview study of children's knowledge about memory. *Monographs of the Society for Research in Child Development, 40*(1, Serial No. 159).

Kreutzer, V.O. (1973). A study of the use of underachieving students as tutors for emotionally disturbed children. *Dissertation Abstracts International, 34*(06-A), 3145.

Krupski, A. (1985). Variations in attention as a function of classroom demands in learning handicapped children. *Early Childhood, 52*(1), 52.

Kuhn, T.S. (1977). A function for thought experiments. In P.N. Johnson-Laird & P.C. Wason (Eds.), *Thinking* (pp. 264–273). New York: Cambridge University Press.

Lamport, K.C. (1982). The effect of inverse tutoring on reading disabled children in a public school setting. *Dissertation Abstracts International, 44*(03-A), 729.

Larson, C.O., Dansereau, D.F., O'Donnell, A.M., Hythecker, V.I., Lambiotte, J.G., & Rocklin, T.R. (1985). Effects of metacognitive and elaborative activity on cooperative learning and transfer. *Contemporary Educational Psychology, 10*, 342–348.

Laughlin, P.R., Branch, L.G., & Johnson, H.H. (1969). Individual versus triadic performance as a function of initial ability. *Journal of Personality and Social Psychology, 12*, 144–150.

Lazerson, D.B. (1980). I must be good if I can teach! – Peer tutoring with aggressive and withdrawn children. *Journal of Learning Disabilities, 13*, 43–48.

Lee, B. (1985). Intellectual origins of Vygotsky's semiotic analysis. In J.V. Wertsch (Ed.), *Culture, communication, and cognition* (pp. 66–93). New York: Cambridge University Press.

Leopold, W.F. (1949). *Speech development of a bilingual child: A linguist's record* (Vol. 3). Evanston, IL: Northwestern University Press.

Liben, L.S. (1987). *Development and learning.* Hillsdale, NJ: Lawrence Erlbaum Associates.

Lillie, D.L. (1975). *Carolina Developmental Profile.* Winston-Salem, NC: Kaplan Press.

Lochhead, J. (1985). Teaching analytic reasoning skills through pair problem solving. In J. Segal, S. Chipman, & R. Glaser (Eds.), *Thinking and learning skills* (Vol. 1, pp. 109–132). Hillsdale, NJ: Lawrence Erlbaum Associates.

Loveland, K.A. (1987). Behavior of young children with Down's syndrome before the mirror: Finding things reflected. *Child Development, 58*(4), 928–936.

Ludeke, R.J., & Hartup, W.W. (1983). Teaching behaviors of 9 and 11-year old girls in mixed-age and same-age dyads. *Journal of Educational Psychology, 75*, 908–914.

Luria, A.R. (1971). Towards the problem of the historical nature of psychological processes. *International Journal of Psychology, 6*, 259–272.

MacMillan, D.L. (1972). Facilitative effect of verbal mediation on paired-associate learning by EMR children. *American Journal of Mental Deficiency, 74*, 611–615.

Maher, C.A. (1984). Handicapped adolescents as cross-age tutors: Program description and evaluation. *Exceptional Children, 51*, 56–63.

Mahoney, G., & Powell, A. (1986). *Transactional intervention with young handicapped children.* Farmington, CT: Pediatric Research and Training Center, University of Connecticut Medical School.

Maier, N.R.F. (1931). Reasoning in humans: II. The solution of a problem and its appearance in consciousness. *Journal of Comparative Psychology, 12,* 181–194.

Mandler, G. (1975). Consciousness: Respectable, useful and probably necessary. In R. Solso (Ed.), *Information processing and cognition: The Loyola Symposium.* Hillsdale, NJ: Lawrence Erlbaum Associates.

Mann, V. (1986). Why some children encounter reading problems: A contribution of difficulties with language processing and phonological sophistication to early reading disability. In J.K. Torgesen & B.Y. Wong (Eds.), *Psychological educational perspectives on learning disabilities* (pp. 133–160). Orlando, FL: Academic Press.

Markoski, B.D. (1983). Conversational interactions of the learning disabled and non-disabled child. *Journal of Learning Disabilities, 16,* 606–609.

Martino, L., & Johnson, D.W. (1979). Cooperative and individualistic experiences among disabled and normal children. *Journal of Social Psychology, 107,* 177–183.

Mayzner, M.S., & Gabriel, R.F. (1963). Information chunking and short-term retention. *Journal of Psychology, 56,* 161–164.

McCarver, R.B. (1972). A developmental study of the effect of organizational cues on short-term memory. *Child Development, 43,* 1317–1325.

McGuire, J., Cherkes-Julkowski, M., & Gertner, N. (1985). *Metacognitive and attributional characteristics of learning disabled, low achieving, and normally achieving junior college students.* Paper presented at the American Educational Research Association, Chicago.

McKinney, J.D. (1973). Problem solving strategies in impulsive and reflective second graders. *Developmental Psychology, 8,* 145.

McKinney, J.D., & Haskins, R. (1980). Cognitive training and the development of problem-solving strategies. *Exceptional Education Quarterly, 1,* 41–51.

McWhorter, K.T., & Levy, J. (1971). The influence of a tutorial program upon tutors. *Journal of Reading, 14,* 221–224.

Mead, G.H. (1934). *Mind, self, and society.* Chicago: University of Chicago Press.

Mervis, C. (1984). Early lexical development: The combinations of mother and child. In C. Sophian (Ed.), *Origins of cognitive skills* (pp. 339–370). Hillsdale, NJ: Lawrence Erlbaum Associates.

Milgram, N.A. (1968). Retention of mediation set in paired-associate learning of normal children and retardates. *Journal of Experimental Child Psychology, 5,* 341–349.

Miller, G.A. (1956). The magical number seven, plus or minus two: Some limitations on our capacity for processing information. *Psychological Review, 63,* 81–87.

Miller, G.A. (1962). *Psychology: The science of mental life.* New York: Harper & Row.

Mondavi, M.S., & Battig, W.F. (1973). Imaginal and verbal mnemonics as related to paired-associate learning and directionality of associations. *Journal of Verbal Learning and Verbal Behavior, 12,* 401–408.

Monoud, P., & Bower, T.G.R. (1975). Conservation of weight in infants. *Cognition, 3,* 29–40.

Montague, M., & Bos, C.S. (1986). The effect of cognitive strategy training on verbal math problem solving performance of learning disabled adolescents. *Journal of Learning Disabilities, 19,* 26–33.

Moynahan, E. (1978). Assessment and selection of paired-associate strategies: A developmental study. *Journal of Experimental Child Psychology, 26,* 257–266.

Mugny, G., & Doise, W. (1978). Socio-cognitive conflict and structuration of individual and collective performances. *European Journal of Social Psychology, 8,* 181–192.

Murphy, L.B. (1974). Coping, vulnerability, and resilience in childhood. In G.V. Coelho,

D.A. Hamberg, & J.E. Adams (Eds.), *Coping and adaptation* (pp. 69–99). New York: Basic Books.

Neimark, E.D., & Slotnick, N.S. (1970). Development of the understanding of logical connectives. *Journal of Educational Psychology, 61*(6), 451–460.

Neisser, U., & Weene, P. (1962). Hierarchies in concept attainment. *Journal of Experimental Psychology, 64*, 640–645.

Nelson, K. (1987). Nativist and functionalist views of cognitive development: Reflections on Keil's review of "Making sense: The acquisition of shared meanings." *Cognitive Development, 2*(3), 237–248.

Nelson, K.E., & Kosslyn, S.M. (1976). Recognition of previously labeled or unlabeled pictures by 5-year-olds and adults. *Journal of Experimental Child Psychology, 21*, 40–45.

Nisbett, R.E., & Bellows, N. (1977). Verbal reports about causal influences of social judgements: Private process versus public theories. *Journal of Personality and Social Psychology, 35*, 613–624.

Nisbett, R.E., & Schachter, S. (1966). Cognitive manipulations of pain. *Journal of Experimental and Social Psychology, 2*, 227–236.

Nisbett, R.E., & Wilson, T.D. (1977). Telling more than we can know: Verbal reports on mental processes. *Psychological Review, 84*, 231–259.

Noel, M.M. (1980). Referential communication abilities of learning disabled children. *Learning Disability Quarterly, 3*, 70–75.

O'Donnell, A.M., Dansereau, D.F., Rocklin, T.R., Hythecker, V.I., Lambiotte, J.G., Larons, C.O., & Young, M.D. (1985). Effects of elaboration frequency on cooperative learning. *Journal of Educational Psychology, 77*, 572–580.

Olsen, D.R. (1976). Culture, technology, and intellect. In L.B. Resnick (Ed.), *The nature of intelligence* (pp. 189–204). New York: John Wiley & Sons.

Olsen, J.L., Wong, B.Y.L., & Marx, R.W. (1983). Linguistic and metacognitive aspects of normally achieving and learning disabled children's communication process. *Learning Disability Quarterly, 6*, 289–304.

Paivio, A. (1971). *Imagery and verbal processes.* New York: Holt, Rinehart, & Winston.

Paivio, A., & Foth, D. (1970). Imaginal and verbal mediators and noun concreteness in paired-associate learning: The elusive interaction. *Journal of Verbal Learning and Verbal Behavior, 9*, 384–390.

Palincsar, A.M., & Brown, A.L. (1984). Reciprocal teaching of comprehension-monitoring activities. *Cognition and Instruction, 1*, 117–175.

Paris, S.G. (1973). Comprehension of language connectives and propositional logical relationships. *Journal of Experimental Psychology, 16*, 278–291.

Paris, S.G., Newman, R.S., & Jacobs, J.E. (1985). Social contexts and functions of children's remembering. In M. Pressley & C.J. Brainerd (Eds.), *Cognitive learning and memory in children.* New York: Springer-Verlag.

Paris, S.G., Newman, R.S., & McVey, K.A. (1982). Learning the functional significance of mnemonic actions: A microgenetic study of strategy acquisition. *Journal of Experimental Child Psychology, 34*, 490–509.

Parmalee, A.J. Jr. (1981). Auditory function and neurological maturation in preterm infants. In S.L. Friedman & M. Sigman (Eds.), *Preterm birth and psychological development.* New York: Academic Press.

Pascual-Leone, J. (1976). On learning and development, Piagetian style: A reply to Lefebvre-Pinard. *Canadian Psychological Review, 17*, 270–289.

Pearl, R., Bryan, T., & Donahue, M. (1980). Learning disabled children's attributions for success and failure. *Learning Disability Quarterly, 3*, 3–9.

Peleg, Z.R., & Moore, R.F. (1982). Effects of the advance organizer with oral and written presentation on recall and inference of EMR adolescents. *American Journal of Mental Deficiency, 86*(6), 621–626.

Perfetti, C., & Hogaboam, T. (1975). Relationship between single word decoding and reading comprehension skills. *Journal of Educational Psychology, 56*, 461–469.

Perret-Clermont, A.N. (1980). *Social interaction and cognitive development in children.* New York: Academic Press.

Peterson, P.L., Janicki, T.C., & Swing, S.R. (1981). Ability × treatment interaction effects on children's learning in large-group and small-group approaches. *American Educational Research Journal, 18*, 453–473.

Piaget, J. (1928). *Judgement and reasoning in the child.* New York: Harcourt Brace.

Piaget, J. (1950). *The psychology of intelligence.* New York: Harcourt Brace.

Piaget, J. (1952). *The origins of intelligence in children.* New York: International Universities' Press.

Piaget, J. (1970). *Structuralism.* New York: Basic Books.

Piaget, J. (1980). *Experiments in contradiction.* Chicago: University of Chicago Press.

Piaget, J., & Inhelder, B. (1969). *The psychology of the child.* New York: Basic Books.

Popper, K.R., & Eccles, J.C. (1977). *The self and its brain, an argument for interactionism.* Boston: Routledge & Kegan Paul.

Pressley, M. (1982). Elaboration and memory development. *Child Development, 53*, 296–309.

Pressley, M., Forrest-Pressley, D., Elliott-Faust, D., & Miller, G. (1985). Children's use of cognitive strategies, how to teach strategies, and what to do if they can't be taught. In M. Pressley & C.J. Brainerd (Eds.), *Cognitive learning and memory in children* (pp. 1–47). New York: Springer-Verlag.

Pressley, M., Levin, J.R., & Ghatala, E.S. (1984). Memory strategy monitoring in adults and children. *Journal of Verbal Learning and Verbal Behavior, 23*, 270–288.

Ratner, H.H. (1984). Memory demands and the development of young children's memory. *Child Development, 55*, 2173–2191.

Raven, J.C. (1958). *Standard progressive matrices.* New York: Psychological Corporation.

Reid, D.K., & Hresko, W. (1981). *A cognitive approach to learning disabilities.* New York: McGraw-Hill.

Roberge, J.J. (1971). An analysis of response patterns for conditional reasoning schemes. *Psychonomic Science, 22*(6), 338–339.

Robinson, J.A., & Kingsley, M.E. (1977). Memory and intelligence: Age and ability differences in strategies and organization of recall. *Intelligence, 1*, 318–330.

Rocissano, L., & Yatchmink, Y. (1983). Language skills and interactive patterns in prematurely born toddlers. *Child Development, 54*, 1229–1241.

Rogoff, B., & Gardner, W. (1984). Adult guidance of cognitive development. In B. Rogoff & J. Lave (Eds.), *Everyday cognition: Its development in social context.* Cambridge, MA: Harvard University Press.

Rosch, E. (1977). Classification of real-world objects: Origin and representations in cognition. In P.N. Johnson-Laird & P.C. Wason (Eds.), *Thinking* (pp. 264–273). New York: Cambridge University Press.

Rosch, E. (1983). Prototype classification and logical classification: The two systems. In E.K. Scholnick (Ed.), *New trends in conceptual representation: Challenges to Piaget's theory?* Hillsdale, NJ: Lawrence Erlbaum Associates.

Rosner, S.R. (1971). The effects of rehearsal and chunking instructions on children's multitrial free recall. *Journal of Experimental Psychology, 11*, 93–105.

Ryugo, D.K., Ryugo, R., Glubus, A., & Killackey, H.P. (1975). Increased spine density in auditory cortex, following visual or somatic differentiation. *Brain Research, 90*, 143–146.

Sabation, D.A. (1983). The house that Jack built. *Journal of Learning Disabilities, 16*, 26–27.

Salatas, H., & Flavell, J. (1976). Retrieval of recently learned information: Development of strategies and control skills. *Child Development, 47*, 941–948.

Sameroff, A. (1982). Development and the dialectic: The need for systems approach. In W.A. Collins (Ed.), *The concept of development, the Minnesota Symposia on Child Psychology* (Vol. 15, pp. 83–104). Hillsdale, NJ: Lawrence Erlbaum Associates.

Sameroff, A.J., & Chandler, M.J. (1975). Reproductive risk and the continuum of caretaking causality. In F.D. Horowitz (Ed.), *Review of child development research* (Vol. 4). Chicago: University of Chicago Press.

Samuels, S.J. (1987). Information processing and reading. *Journal of Learning Disabilities, 20*, 18–22.

Schiffrin, R.M., & Dumais, S. (1981). The development of automatism. In J.K. Anderson (Ed.), *Cognitive skills and their acquisition* (pp. 111–140). Hillsdale, NJ: Lawrence Erlbaum Associates.

Scribner, W., & Cole, M. (1973). Cognitive consequences of formal and informal education. *Science, 182*, 553–559.

Scruggs, T.E., Mastropieri, M.A., & Richter, L. (1985). Peer tutoring with behaviorally disordered students: Social and academic benefits. *Behavioral Disorders, 10*(4), 283–294.

Scruggs, T.E., & Richter, L. (1986). Tutoring learning disabled students: A critical review. *Learning Disability Quarterly, 9*, 2–14.

Shapiro, B.J., & O'Brien, T. (1970). Logical thinking in children ages six through sixteen. *Child Development, 41*, 823–829.

Shapiro, S.I., & Moely, B.E. (1971). Free recall, subjective organization, and learning to learn at three age levels. *Psychonomic Science, 23*, 189–190.

Sharan, S. (1980). Cooperative learning in small groups: Recent methods and effects on achievement, attitudes, and ethnic relations. *Review of Educational Research, 50*, 241–272.

Shatz, M., & Gelman, R. (1973). The development of communication skills: Modifications in the speech of young children as a function of the listener. *Monographs of the Society for Research in Child Development*, Serial No. 152, 38.

Shepherd, M.J., Gelzheiser, L.M., & Solar, R.A. (1984). *Cross-age investigations of learning disabled and non-disabled children's spontaneous use of mnemonic strategies* (Tech. Rep. No. 32). New York: Research Institute for the Study of Learning Disabilities, Teachers' College, Columbia University.

Sherman, S.M. (1977). The effect of cortical and tectal lesions on the visual fields of binocularly deprived cats. *Journal of Comparative Neurology, 172*, 231–246.

Shweder, R.A. (1977). Likeness and Likelihood in everyday thought: magical thinking and everyday judgments about personality. In P.N. Johnson-Laird & P.C. Wason (Eds.), *Thinking*. NY: Cambridge University Press.

Siegler, R.S. (1978). The origins of scientific reasoning. In R. Siegler (Ed.), *Children's thinking: What develops?* (pp. 109–150). New York: John Wiley & Sons.

Silverman, I.W., & Geiringer, E. (1973). Dyadic interaction and conservation induction: A test of Piaget's equilibration model. *Child Development, 44,* 815–820.

Silverman, I.W., & Stone, J.M. (1972). Modifying cognitive functioning through participation in a problem-solving group. *Journal of Educational Psychology, 63,* 603–608.

Sindelar, P.T. (1982). The effects of hypothesis/test and fluency training, cross-age tutoring, and small group instruction, on reading skills. *Dissertation Abstracts International, 38*(10), 6060.

Skon, L., Johnson, D.W., & Johnson, R.T. (1981). Cooperative peer interaction versus individual competition and individualistic efforts: Effects on the acquisition of cognitive reasoning strategies. *Journal of Educational Psychology, 73,* 83–92.

Slavin, R.E. (1978). Effects of student teams and peer tutoring on academic achievement and time on task. *Journal of Experimental Education, 48,* 252–257.

Smith, C. (1979). Children's understanding of natural hierarchies. *Journal of Experimental Child Psychology, 27,* 437–458.

Smith, E.R., & Miller, F.D. (1978). Limits on perception of cognitive processes: A reply to Nisbett and Wilson. *Psychological Review, 85,* 355–362.

Smith, K., Johnson, D., & Johnson, R. (1981). Can conflict be constructive? Controversy versus concurrence seeking in learning groups. *Journal of Educational Psychology, 73,* 651–663.

Snyder, M., Schulz, R., & Jones, E.E. (1974). Expectancy and apparent duration as determinants of fatigue. *Journal of Personality and Social Psychology, 29,* 426–434.

Soensken, P.A., Flagg, C.L., & Schmits, D.W. (1981). Social communication in learning disabled students: A pragmatic analysis. *Journal of Learning Disabilities, 14,* 283–286.

Spekman, N.J. (1981). Dyadic verbal communication abilities of learning disabled and normally achieving fourth and fifth-grade boys. *Learning Disability Quarterly, 4,* 139–151.

Spitz, H.H. (1966). The role of input organization in the learning and memory of mental retardates. In N.R. Ellis (Ed.), *International review of research in mental retardation* (Vol. 2, pp. 29–56). New York: Academic Press.

Spurlin, J.E., Dansereau, D.F., Larson, D.O., & Brooks, L.W. (1984). Cooperative learning strategies in processing descriptive text: Effects of role and activity level of the learner. *Cognition and Instruction, 1,* 451–463.

Stanford, A.R. (1978). *Learning accomplishment profile.* Winston-Salem, NC: Kaplan Press.

Stein, B. (1977). The effect of cue-target uniqueness on cued recall performance. *Memory & Cognition, 5,* 319–322.

Steinberg, Z.D., & Cazden, C.B. (1979). Children as teachers—of peer and ourselves. *Theory and Practice, 18,* 258–266.

Stern, M., & Hildebrandt, K.A. (1986). Prematurity steroryping: Effects on mother–infant interaction. *Child Development, 57*(2), 308–315.

Sternberg, R.J., & Wagner, R.K. (1982). Automization failure in learning disabilities. *Topics in Learning and Learning Disabilities, 2,* 1–11.

Stolzenberg, J.B., & Cherkes-Julkowski, M. (1987). *Attention deficit hyperactivity disorder—A problem of learning and living.* Paper presented at the 17th Annual State Conference of the Association for Children and Adults with Learning Disabilities, Hartford, CT.

Stone, C.A., & Wertsch, J.V. (1984). A social interactional analysis of learning disabilities remediation. *Journal of Learning Disabilities, 17,* 194–199.

Storms, M.D., & Nisbett, R.E. (1970). Insomnia and the attribution process. *Journal of Personality and Social Psychology*, *2*, 319–328.

Strauss, A.A., & Lehtinen, L.E. (1947). *Psychopathology and education of brain-injured children*. New York: Grune & Stratton.

Strauss, M.S., & Curtis, L.E. (1981). Infant perception of numerosity. *Child Development*, *52*(4), 1146–1152.

Strauss, M.S., & Curtis, L.E. (1984). Development of numerical concepts in infancy. In C. Sophian (Ed.), *Origins of cognitive skills* (pp. 131–156). Hillsdale, NJ: Lawrence Erlbaum Associates.

Strauss, S. (1982). *U-shaped behavioral growth*. New York: Academic Press.

Swanson, H.L. (1987). Information processing theory and learning disabilities: A commentary and future perspective. *Journal of Learning Disabilities*, *20*(3), 155–166.

Swing, S.R., & Peterson, P.L. (1982). The relationship of student ability and small-group interaction to student achievement. *American Educational Research Journal*, *19*, 257–274.

Taplin, J.E. (1971). Reasoning with conditional sentences. *Journal of Verbal Learning and Verbal Behavior*, *10*, 219–225.

Taplin, J.E., & Staudenmeyer, H. (1973). Interpretation of abstract conditional sentences in deductive reasoning. *Journal of Verbal Learning and Verbal Behavior*, *12*, 530–542.

Taylor, A.M., & Turnure, J.E. (1979). Imagery and verbal elaboration with retarded children: Effects on learning and memory. In N.R. Ellis (Ed.), *Handbook of mental deficiency, psychological theory, and research* (2nd ed., pp. 659–698). Hillsdale, NJ: Lawrence Erlbaum Associates.

Tees, R.C. (1979). The effect of visual deprivation on pattern recognition in the rat. *Developmental Psychobiology*, *12*, 485–497.

Tenney, Y.J. (1975). The child's conception of organization and recall. *Journal of Experimental Child Psychology*, *19*, 100–114.

Thelen, E. (1986). Treadmill elicited stepping in seven-month-old infants. *Child Development*, *57*(6), 1498–1506.

Thoman, E.B. (1987). Self-regulation of stimulation by prematures with a Breathing Blue Bear. In J.J. Gallagher & C.T. Ramey (Eds.), *The malleability of children* (pp. 51–70). Baltimore: Brookes Publishing.

Thorndike, R.L., Hagen, E.P., & Sattler, J.M. (1986). *Stanford–Binet Intelligence Scale* (4th Ed.). Chicago: Riverside Publishing Company.

Torgesen, J.K. (1980). Implications of the LD child's use of efficient task strategies. *Journal of Learning Disabilities*, *13*(7), 364–371.

Torgesen, J.K. (1982). The learning disabled child as an inactive learner: Educational implications. *Topics in Learning and Learning Disabilities*, *2*(1), 45–52.

Torgesen, J.K., & Goldman, T. (1977). Verbal rehearsal and short-term memory in reading disabled children. *Child Development*, *48*, 56–60.

Torgesen, J.K., & Licht, B.G. (1983). The learning disabled as an inactive learner: Retrospect and prospects. In D. McKinney & L. Feagans (Eds.), *Current topics in learning disabilities* (Vol. 1, pp. 3–31). Norwood, NJ: Ablex.

Torgesen, J.K., Murphy, H., & Ivey, C. (1979). The effects of an orienting task on the memory performance of reading disabled children. *Journal of Learning Disabilities*, *12*, 396–401.

Turner, L.A., & Bray, N.W. (1985). Spontaneous rehearsal by mildly mentally retarded children and adolescents. *American Journal of Mental Deficiency*, *90*(1), 57–63.

Turnure, J.E., & Thurlow, M.L. (1973). Verbal elaboration and the promotion of transfer of training in educable mentally retarded children. *Journal of Experimental Child Psychology, 15*, 137–148.

Uzgiris, I.C., & Hunt, J.M. (1975). *Assessment in infancy, Ordinal Scales of Psychological Development*. Chicago: University of Illinois Press.

Uzgiris, I.C., & Hunt, J.M. (1987). *Infant performance and experience: New findings with the Ordinal Scales*. Chicago: University of Illinois Press.

Vellutino, F.R., & Steger, J.A. (1975). Verbal vs non-verbal paired-associates learning in poor and normal readers. *Neuropsychologia, 13*, 75–82.

Vygotsky, L.S. (1962). *Thought and language*. Cambridge, MA: MIT Press.

Vygotsky, L.S. (1978). Internalization of higher psychological functions. In M. Cole, V. John-Steiner, S. Scritmer, & E. Souberman (Eds.), *Mind in society: The development of higher psychological processes* (pp. 52–57). Cambridge, MA: Harvard University Press.

Vygotsky, L.S. (1981). The genesis of higher level functions. In J.V. Wertsch (Eds.), *The concept of activity in Soviet psychology*. Armonk, NY: Sharpe.

Wachs, T.D. (1985). Toys as an aspect of the physical environment: Constraints and nature of relationship to development. *Topics in Early Childhood Special Education, 5*(3), 31–46.

Wallace, J.G. (1982). An information processing viewpoint on monotone assessment of monotone development. In S. Strauss (Eds.), *U-shaped behavioral growth* (pp. 87–100). New York: Academic Press.

Wanschura, P.B., & Borkowski, J.G. (1975). Long-term transfer of a mediational strategy by moderately retarded children. *American Journal of Mental Deficiency, 80*, 323–333.

Wason, P.C. (1972). Self contradictions. In P.N. Johnson-Laird & P.C. Wason (Eds.), *Thinking* (pp. 114–128). New York: Cambridge University Press.

Wason, P.C., & Johnson-Laird, P.N. (1972a). *Psychology of reasoning*. Cambridge, MA: Harvard University Press.

Wason, P.C., & Johnson-Laird, P.N. (1972b). *Thinking*. New York: Cambridge University Press.

Waters, H.S. (1982). Memory development during adolescence: Relationship between metamemory, strategy use, and performance. *Journal of Experimental Child Psychology, 33*, 183–195.

Watson, G.B. (1928). Do groups think more efficiently than individuals? *Journal of Abnormal and Social Psychology, 23*, 328–336.

Webb, N.M. (1980). A process-outcome analysis of learning in group and individual settings. *Educational Psychologist, 15*, 69–83.

Webb, N.M. (1982). Student interaction and learning in small groups. *Review of Educational Research, 52*(3), 421–445.

Wechsler, D.I. (1974). *Wechsler Intelligence Scale for Children—Revised*. New York: Psychological Corporation.

Weiner, B. (1974). *Achievement motivation and attribution theory*. Morristown, NJ: General Learning Press.

Weir, R.H., & Venezky, R.L. (1968). Spelling-to-sound patterns. In K.S. Goodman (Ed.), *The psycholinguistic nature of the reading process*. Detroit: Wayne State University Press.

Wellman, H.M. (1977). The early development of intentional memory behavior. *Human Development, 20*, 86–101.

Wellman, H.M. (1985). The origins of metacognition. In D.L. Forrest-Pressley, G.E. MacKinnon, & T.G. Waller (Eds.), *Metacognition, cognition, and human performance* (pp. 1–31). New York: Academic Press.

Wertsch, J., McNamee, G., Budwig, N., & McLane, J. (1980). The adult–child dyad as a problem-solving system. *Child Development, 51*, 1215–1221.

Wertsch, J.V., Minick, N., & Arns, F.J. (1984). The creation of context in joint problem-solving. In B. Rogoff & J. Lave (Eds.), *Everyday cognition: Its development in social context.* Cambridge, MA: Harvard University Press.

Whimbey, A., & Lochhead, J. (1980). *Problem solving and comprehension: A short course in analytical reasoning.* Philadelphia: Franklin Institute Press.

Whimbey, A., & Lochhead, J. (1981). *Developing mathematical skills: Computation, problem solving, and basics for algebra.* New York: McGraw-Hill.

Wickelgren, W.A. (1967). Rehearsal, grouping, and hierarchical organization of serial position cues in short-term memory. *Quarterly Journal of Experimental Psychology, 19*, 97–102.

Wishart, J.G. (1987). Performance of young nonretarded children and children with Down's syndrome on Piagetian infant search tasks. *American Journal of Mental Deficiency, 92*(2), 169–177.

Witelson, S.F. (1977). Early hemisphere specialization and interhemispheric plasticity: An empirical and theoretical review. In S.J. Segalowitz & F.A. Gruber (Eds.), *Language development and neurological theory.* New York: Academic Press.

Witelson, S.F. (1987). Neurobiological aspects of language in children. *Child Development, 58*(3), 653–688.

Wolff, P., & Levin, J.R. (1972). The role of overt activity in children's imagery production. *Child Development, 43*, 537–547.

Wong, B. (1980). Activating the inactive learner: Use of questions/prompts to enhance comprehension and retention of implied information in learning disabled children. *Learning Disability Quarterly, 3*(1), 29–37.

Wong, B., Wong, R., & Foth, D. (1977). Recall and clustering of verbal materials among normal and poor readers. *Bulletin of the Psychonomic Society, 10*, 375–377.

Wood, D., Bruner, J.S., & Ross, G. (1976). The role of tutoring in problem solving. *Journal of Child Psychology and Psychiatry, 17*, 89–100.

Wood, D., & Middleton, D. (1975). A study of assisted problem solving. *British Journal of Psychology, 66*, 181–191.

Yarrow, L.J., Rubenstein, J.L., & Pederson, F.A. (1975). *Infant and environment: Early cognitive and motivational development.* New York: John Wiley & Sons.

Yuille, J.C., & Paivio, A. (1968). Imagery and verbal mediation instructions in paired-associate learning. *Journal of Experimental Psychology, 78*, 436–441.

Zadeh, L.A. (1982). A note on prototype theory and fuzzy sets. *Cognition, 12*, 291–297.

Zaidel, E. (1979). Performance on the ITPA following cerebral commissurotomy and hemispherectomy. *Neuropsychologia, 17*(3–4), 259–280.

Zeaman, D., & House, B.J. (1963). The role of attention in retardate discrimination learning. In N.R. Ellis (Ed.), *International review of research in mental retardation* (Vol. 2). New York: Academic Press.

Zeaman, D., & House, B.J. (1979). A review of attention theory. In N.R. Ellis (Ed.) *Handbook of mental deficiency, psychological theory, and research* (pp. 63–120). Hillsdale, NJ: Lawrence Erlbaum Associates.

Zelazo, P.R. (1982). The year-old infant: A period of major cognitive change. In T.G. Bever (Ed.), *Regression in mental development—Basic phenomena and theories* (pp. 47–80). Hillsdale, NJ: Lawrence Erlbaum Associates.

Zimmerman, B.J., & Blom, D.E. (1983). On resolving conflicting views of cognitive conflict. *Developmental Review, 3*, 62–72.

Author Index

Subject Index